R E V I E W S

Dr. High's book provides important insights for people both in the lay public and medical professions to better understand the differences in heart disease in women versus their male counterparts. The information is very well organized, evidence based, and easy to understand. As coronary artery disease prevalence is on the rise in females world-wide and is the #1 killer in the U.S., Dr. High is providing an important social service by bringing this issue to the public forefront.

— **Sandeep Rajan Singh, M.D.**, *Cardiologist*

As a Professor for Health Promotion and an advocate in community health education specializing in self-disease detection and prevention, I found Dr. High's book to be a beaming spotlight that shines on the misconceptions of the top killer of women in the United States, heart disease. More often, women believe that this is a "male" medical issue and therefore are not aware of taking precautionary measures to offset heart disease, much less recognize the signs of heart disease that may differ drastically than symptoms males may experience.

I plan on making Dr. High's book mandatory reading for my students to assist them in becoming better health educators and health care providers. Her approach is easily comprehendible for all readers, provides the urgency that is needed for attention, and is all-comprehensive for heart health issues in women from A to Z.

— **Erin K. O'Neill, PhD, CHES, CSCS**, *Professor: New Jersey City University Department of Health Sciences*

Arguably the most important asset for women to have in their arsenal against the number one killer, Dr. High's book is now securely in the hands of my daughters and granddaughters.

— **Shirley Valentine**, *Retired*

Women's health is receiving well-deserved attention in this book, especially with symptoms being different than men. It's a great detail for the general public to start getting educated not only for getting treated in a timely fashion but also prevention of cardiovascular disease.

As a Medical Oncologist, I could not agree more about prevention and early treatment of heart disease in women. Both cancer and heart disease being competitive Killers in Women, this book comes highly recommended.

— **Harman Kaur, M.D.**, *Medical Oncologist*

This book clearly delivers the fact that heart disease kills more women than breast cancer. As women we might want to add a red ribbon to our lapels along with the pink one we currently wear.

— **Wendy Jenkins**, *Vice President, Leisure and Recreation Concepts, Inc.*

This is a book that all women should read. It answers not only the questions that may be known but also the questions that should be asked. Dr. High uses simple language to answer complicated questions that any women can understand and literally "take to heart." Dr. High is truly concerned about women's health and has taken the courage to make it her priority to help all women understand their own health. Every woman should read this book if not only to understand the importance of learning about their own heart health but maybe to help a mother, sister, or daughter become more aware as well.

— **Susan Winborn Fullerton**, *Registered Pharmacist*

Living in a small rural town with the closest cardiologist 50 miles away, I found this book full of helpful information, and it provides valuable assistance and direction for women of ALL ages. It's a great New Year's resolution book!

—**Jana Trotter**, *Community Volunteer & Fundraiser*

This is an easy to read book by a leading female cardiologist that puts the fear of women's biggest health problem into layman terms. It allows readers to feel they are discussing their health with their cardiologist with statistics and data to help them understand their risk and options and benefits of treatment. I will use it in my clinical practice to put my patients at ease.

—**Melissa M. Carry, M.D. FACC**, *Fellow of the American College of Cardiology & Staff Cardiologist, Baylor Hospital, Dallas*

Dr. High writes in such a conversational style about a subject that most women, including my girlfriends, never discuss. Heart disease and prevention should be included in every "Girls Night Out" conversation along with clothes, shoes, and men! Love yourself and your girls (or friends). Dr. High is definitely THE voice for women's health.

—**Tara Thomas**, *Sommelier*

Why Most Women Die

How Women Can Fight Their #1 Killer: Heart Disease

Shyla T. High, M.D.

Stay heclthy!!

Shyla T. High

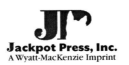

Jackpot Press, Inc.
A Wyatt-MacKenzie Imprint

Why Most Women Die
How Women Can Fight Their #1 Killer: Heart Disease
Shyla T. High, M.D.

ISBN: 978-1-939288-02-8
Library of Congress Control Number: 2012953630

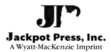

Jackpot Press, Inc.
A Wyatt-MacKenzie Imprint

Published by Jackpot Press, Inc., A Wyatt-MacKenzie Imprint
jackpotpress@wyattmackenzie.com

Cover Photo: Chris Pittman, Pittman Photography.
Proofreading: Karen Kibler
Index: Jean Jesensky, Endswell Indexing
Medical Illustrations by Megan Rojas, medicalillustrator.com

www.WhyMostWomenDie.com

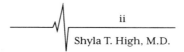

Shyla T. High, M.D.

Table of Contents

About the Author   iv

Introduction   v

1 The Coming Tsunami   1

2 Are you at risk?   11

3 Heal Thyself   29

4 Symptoms and Tests   37

5 So if it's Not a Heart Attack, What is It?   49

6 So You're Having a Heart Attack   58

7 To Take or Not to Take: The Skinny on Meds   71

8 Sex, Suds, Supplements, and Stress   85

9 Other Heart Conditions   95

10 Leftovers   105

Appendix   115

Index   117

ABOUT THE AUTHOR

A practicing general cardiologist since 1998, Shyla T. High, M.D., is Board Certified by the American College of Cardiology and is the current North East District chair of the Texas Club of Internists. A frequent guest speaker, Dr. High has a particular interest in women's heart health, recognizing the seriousness of the impending heart disease epidemic and the urgent need to take proactive steps to avoid it. Prior to medical school she was a practicing pharmacist for eight years. Dr. High currently practices and resides in Dallas, Texas.

INTRODUCTION

For some reason, my father, a successful attorney, always felt that I had the gifts and talents for a career in medicine. Maybe even the kind of career that can make a real difference. And although I liked the science, the idea of actually seeing patients and having to deal with sick people all day long just wasn't anything I found appealing. I became a pharmacist instead. I enjoyed it and felt a real sense of satisfaction from the work. My life was all set.

Then one day, at the age of 29, I received a phone call from my mother. My father was headed to the hospital for observation after experiencing chest pain. Within 48 hours, my father was dead. He was just 58.

Within three months I found myself closing my pharmacy practice and answering a call to enter the medical profession. Maybe it was to make sense of my father's death. Maybe it was to follow his original instincts about my career path. Whatever it was, it seemed powerfully right. And so while my friends were all settling into their careers and starting families, I went back to square one. I applied to medical school. It was a step backward, but I had a strong sense that it would eventually result in a big step forward.

Medical school ultimately led to cardiology and in 1998, I began my practice. In the years since, I've regained that sense of satisfaction I had with my pharmacy. My new career really was a big step forward. I've helped people. But I've also come to understand that there is much to be done, more than can be done in a single practice. Cardiovascular disease continues to claim the lives of hundreds of thousands of people each year across the United States. More disturbing is the trend towards its claim on women. It's no longer a man's disease. Today, in fact, more women are dying of heart disease than men.

Hence, this book. The tide of cardiovascular disease needs to be turned. But to accomplish that, we need to do it one life—one heart—at a time. Such is how differences are made. I'd like to start with you. If you've picked up this book, chances are you're concerned about your heart health and you're looking for some simple, straightforward information. I'm confident you'll find it in here.

You might find some sobering statistics, too. For me, the matter of women's heart health went from serious, as I began writing this book, to urgent the deeper I went. What I initially assumed was a call for good, solid information on women's heart health, became, in my mind, a burning need. The more I researched, the more imperative it became for me

Shyla T. High, M.D.

to finish this book. The stakes are high, higher than I had realized. Women are dying and way too little is being said or done about it.

I hope to be a voice that might help change that. I hope to educate and I hope to at least start a dialogue. Get people talking about the seriousness of cardiovascular disease with respect to women. On an individual level, I hope to help you.

And somewhere in all of this, I hope to prove my dad's instincts right.

Shyla T. High, MD.

CHAPTER ONE

The Coming Tsunami

The Disconnect

It's a major threat to women. The biggest health threat of all, in fact. Nothing poses more of a risk. More than a third of deaths in American women over the age of twenty are caused by it. Over 400,000 women will die of it in the United States alone this year—over 1,000 per day, about one death every 78 seconds.

Yet there are relatively few ribbons being worn for it, few awareness campaigns, few fundraising events, few charity drives, few walkathons. Cardiovascular disease remains in the shadows. But the fact is, CVD kills more women than all forms of cancer *combined*.

Another surprising fact: cardiovascular disease kills more women than men. And yet cardiovascular disease is still considered "a man's disease." Certainly there was a time when it was. Up until 1984, the majority of heart attack deaths were men. The prototypical (almost stereotypical) heart attack victim was the breadwinning, stressed-out, male business executive. But those days are gone, replaced by a whole different dynamic on the health front. The tables have now turned. An estimated 42 million American women now live with cardiovascular disease. And more women than men will die within one year of having a heart attack. Of the survivors, more women than men will develop congestive heart failure within five years and will have more complications resulting from bypass surgeries.

African-American women are twice as likely to be at risk for heart disease as white women, with higher rates of obesity, high cholesterol, and high blood pressure. In fact, more African-American women die of heart disease than any other group of Americans. Hispanic-American women are at greater risk than white women as well with almost a third of Mexican-American women having CVD, according to the American Heart Association. But very rapidly, cardiovascular disease seems to be cutting across all ethnic lines.

Here's the disconnect: According to a recent poll by the American Heart Association, only 13% of women recognize that CVD is, in fact, their most

Shyla T. High, M.D.

serious health threat. 87% of women cite cancer (particularly breast), or some other disease as presenting more of a danger.

Unrecognized

What's more surprising is that the news of CVD's furtive encroachment into the female camp isn't fully recognized even by many within the medical community. Women's health issues can be more complex than men's and sometimes doctors might simply overlook the risks of heart disease with their female patients. Fortunately, this is beginning to change as awareness within the medical community continues to grow, but often times CVD is still thought of, even by health care providers, as a man's disease. And it's a man's disease treated by men. Only a meager 8% of cardiologists are women.

The coupling of these factors—a doctor not thinking in terms of CVD with a female patient and the patient not appropriately concerned either—is a dangerous mix. What makes it even more dangerous is the fact that symptoms of heart disease are often different in women than the classic symptoms we've come to associate with the disease, at least as they manifest themselves in men. This means that women are more likely to delay getting treatment, not recognizing their problem as heart-related. If that isn't bad enough, once they do seek medical help, the attending *doctor* might not even recognize the symptoms. So not only is CVD in women going unrecognized as a sort of macro, societal problem, it's sometimes not even recognized at the individual level when a woman is having a serious heart event.

All of this is not necessarily anyone's fault. It's a simple matter of awareness, or lack thereof. Where symptoms are concerned, for example, we've been conditioned, inside and outside of the medical community, to expect chest pain and yet chest pain isn't always present when a woman is having a heart attack. It's not always present when a man is having a heart attack either, but it's a symptom that, with men, is less likely to be absent. And so when a woman seeks treatment for, say, indigestion and extreme fatigue—but no chest pain—the idea that she might be having a heart attack might be overlooked, even though her apparent symptoms might say otherwise to the astute medical professional. It's a critical point; when a younger woman is having a heart attack, and chest pain is not part of the equation, she is 20% more likely to die than a male.

Conversely, just to complicate things, when chest pain is present in women, it doesn't always mean a heart attack. With women, there's a higher incidence of chest pain that is not related to the

Shyla T. High, M.D.

heart. It could be stress or any number of other things, including pleurisy, muscle strain, or maybe just heartburn.

Mindsets

Women are slower to seek treatment, too, and that doesn't help the numbers. Most of it is due to the awareness factor. But some of it is just due to the female mindset. Even if there's some level of recognition of the onset of a serious heart event, a woman might be more likely to downplay its significance. Women are the caregivers. Multi-taskers. Generally tougher and with a higher tolerance for pain. We're busy. We work all day and take the kids to soccer practice and make dinner. People are counting on us. We don't have time to have heart attacks! And besides, our doctors haven't discussed heart disease with us, so what's the big deal? It's a man's disease, after all.

This mindset delays the trip to the hospital, the hospital delays treatment by seeking other causes for the patient's symptoms, and frequently real damage occurs if not outright tragedy. What's most tragic is this: 75% of heart disease is preventable, but it's not being prevented. Three out of four women who have heart disease shouldn't have it. Of course therein lies the good news. If the mindset changes, if serious symptoms are recognized for what they are, if women understand the risks, if the medical profession jumps on board, collectively, we can reduce cardiovascular disease by 75%.

The alternative is almost too terrible to contemplate. The risk of CVD increases as one gets older and the statistics are only going to become more frightening as the baby boom population ages. More than 50 million women are now over 50 years old. The situation could become grim. With close to one out of two women at risk of dying of heart attack and stroke, we're facing the leading edge of a catastrophic tsunami.

Dangerous Trends

How did we get here? Why the increase in risk of CVD among women? Some of it has to do with today's more sedentary lifestyle, some of it has to do with poorer eating habits. Our grandmothers and great-grandmothers were generally more active and ate healthier. Our creature comforts and higher standard of living mean we lead less physically-demanding lives. As women, we're in the workplace more today, too—sitting at desks, sitting behind computers. The key word is sitting. We try exercise programs but more often than not, we don't stick to them. Studies show we eat more (a lot more) and the foods we eat today are more highly-processed type foods and often contain higher concentrations of sodium and fat. We try dieting, but, as with exercising, we don't always stick with our diets either.

Both relative lack of physical activity and poor dietary habits are highlighted by this incontrovertible piece of evidence: over one-third of Americans are now considered obese. Not just overweight, mind you, but obese.

Naturally, these trends transcend gender. Men as well as women are more obese in today's America than yesterday's. (The percentage of obese Americans was just 13% in 1960!) And so the prevalence of heart disease is up for everybody. The number ten killer in the country at the start of the twentieth century, heart disease is now number one. Consequently, the increase in CVD among women can be explained at least in part by the increase overall. But another factor is directly related to women: more women begin smoking at a younger age than men. And less women than men are inclined to quit as they get older. Worse, recent studies seem to indicate that smoking presents a higher risk of heart disease for women than it does for men, maybe as much as 25% higher. For some reason, smoking seems to be more potent for women.[1] Smoking, as it turns out, is a great way to take yourself down the path towards cardiovascular disease.

[1]"Increased risk of coronary heart disease in female smokers", Mark Woodward, Rachel R Huxley, The Lancet, 3 March 2012 [Vol. 379, Issue 9818, Page 803]

Becoming Aware

But perhaps the biggest explanation for the increase in CVD in women gets us back to the simplest explanation: lack of awareness, both by women themselves and by the medical community in general. Men have been conditioned for decades to be concerned about their hearts; doctors have been conditioned for decades to be concerned right along with them. Women, on the other hand simply don't think in those terms, nor, unfortunately, do a lot of their doctors. And with lack of awareness comes lack of prevention. Simply put, we're seeing an increase in CVD among women because we're just not doing enough to stop it.

The key to heading off the potential tsunami is to get women thinking about heart health. To do that, we all—women and medical providers both—have to not only start paying attention to the issue, but to think differently about it than how we think about it where men are concerned. Yes, the symptoms of a heart event are often different but the factors of heart disease are also often different with women. There are hormonal factors, for example. There are different risks. There are different considerations for treatment. It's not enough, in other words, to think about the heart. We have to think about the female heart in particular and all of the elements that come along with it. Women are different than men, after all. That's no surprise. So it shouldn't be surprising that female heart health is different than male heart health.

Here's the big picture: the history of female heart disease around the world tells us that it's not a natural condition. That its prevalence has increased so significantly just in the past twenty or thirty years, tells us that it's not something necessarily inherent in the human condition. It's a relatively new trend. And trends by their very nature can be reversed. If CVD is not a natural condition, then we can push it back. We just need to understand how. We're probably never going to be able to completely eradicate cardiovascular disease from the face of the earth, but if we know how to prevent at least 75% of it, then we can put a pretty big dent in it.

Getting Started

It's one thing, of course, to try to get one's head around the issue of CVD in the aggregate sense—how it affects women in general, how it, in turn, affects our society, etc. But let's leave that for the medical profession. It's a big issue that hopefully will soon start being recognized as such. But my hunch is that slowing down the potential tsunami is the kind of thing that we're going to have to do on a person by person basis, one woman at a time.

Maybe we can start with you. If you're alarmed by the statistics and concerned about your own heart health, you should be. But there's no reason to panic. You may not even be at risk. But let's make sure. If you are at risk, let's find out how to minimize it. Together, let's take the necessary steps towards maintaining a healthy heart. If awareness is the first step, then educating yourself about your heart health is the second.

Pulse Points

- More than a third of deaths in American women over the age of twenty are caused by heart disease.

- Cardiovascular disease kills more women than all forms of cancer combined.

- When chest pain, the traditional symptom of a heart attack, isn't present, a woman is 20% more likely to die than a man.

- The percentage of obese Americans was 13% in 1960. Now, almost one out of three American are obese.

- 75% of heart disease is preventable!

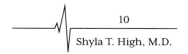

CHAPTER TWO

Are you at risk?

Heart Disease Defined

What does it mean to be at risk for heart disease? What, more fundamentally, do we even mean by "heart disease"? In its most basic sense, heart disease is when plaque (essentially fat and cholesterol, along with calcium and a few other substances) builds up in the arteries of the heart causing a dangerous thickening of the artery walls. Plaque buildup in general terms is technically called atherosclerosis, or atherosclerotic vascular disease, and can happen anywhere in the body. When it happens in the heart, it's called *cardio*vascular disease (CVD)—cardio meaning heart—or we might just refer to it simply as heart disease. If a person has heart disease, it may mean vascular disease elsewhere, too, increasing the chance of stroke.

Plaque buildup is largely asymptomatic—you won't feel anything that tells you the plaque is building up—until about 75% of the artery becomes blocked. Then the blockage may produce symptoms that can mimic a heart attack, though to a less intense degree, typically doing so when the heart is under stress (physical exertion, for example). A person may feel chest pain, termed angina pectoris or simply angina. If the plaque buildup gets to the point where about 90% of the artery is blocked, a person can experience angina even at rest.

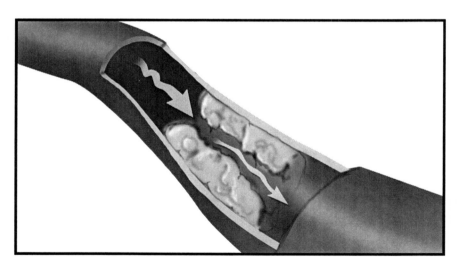

ILLUSTRATION 1. **BLOCKED ARTERY**

Shyla T. High, M.D.

A heart attack is when the artery becomes 100% blocked, normally as the result of a blood clot fully obstructing an artery already significantly blocked by plaque. A heart attack is angina that lasts longer, is typically more intense, and is usually accompanied by other symptoms such as sweating, nausea, or radiating pain in the upper extremities or jaw. With a heart attack, the lack of blood begins to kill the heart muscle which quickly becomes electrically unstable; the rhythm is disrupted and the situation quickly becomes life threatening.

Interestingly, clots are formed by the body as a response to bodily trauma—as a way for the body to repair itself, in other words. If blood didn't coagulate (clot), we'd bleed to death if cut. But in cases of heart disease, the blood might coagulate as a response to a damaged arterial wall, or maybe because it's been rendered stagnant by the buildup of plaque. A heart attack is when a good thing (a bodily repair technique, i.e. a clot) goes terribly bad. The question is, how do you stop it from happening?

Know the Risks

Why do some people experience plaque buildup and the resultant narrowing of their arteries while others don't? What contributes to plaque buildup? How can it be avoided? Are *you* at risk?

The risk factors for heart disease can be divided into two basic categories—modifiable and non-modifiable. Non-modifiable risks include age and genetic factors. If you have a family history of heart disease—in particular, a primary male relative (parent or sibling) with heart disease under the age of 55, or a primary female relative (parent or sibling) with heart disease under the age of 65—you may be predisposed to heart disease yourself. And it's no surprise that people are more prone to heart disease as they age. An 80-year-old has had 60 more years of potential plaque buildup than a 20-year-old. Women tend to lag behind men by about ten years when it comes to the clinical presentation of heart disease with age. The body's production of estrogen provides a natural protection for women in a pre-menopausal state (at least absent other—modifiable—risks). All bets are off, though, post-menopause. At that point, we catch up to men and catch up quickly.

There's not much we can do about the non-modifiable risks (hence their name). We can't help what family we're born into and there's only one sure-fire alternative to getting older and it's not a very attractive one. If we're predisposed genetically to heart disease, we just need to pay a little more attention to our bodies. We need to do the same as we age. We need to minimize the risks by managing those things we *can* control.

And that brings us to the modifiable factors:

- Smoking
- Obesity
- Physical Inactivity
- Blood Pressure
- Cholesterol
- Diabetes

Lighting Up

Of course, some of our risk factors overlap. Some of them lead to others. Physical inactivity can lead to obesity, for example. The wrong diet can lead to high cholesterol. These factors are dangerous enough taken individually. Added together, they become much, much worse.

All of them are modifiable. Yes, some, like obesity, can have genetic components, but they're all basically tied to lifestyle choices. And that's the good news. The operative word is "choices." We can minimize these risks simply by choosing to do so.

If I had to pick the one that's the most dangerous risk factor, the one above all the rest, the most lethal one, the selection would be easy: smoking. Smoking is the number one preventable cause of death in the world. A lot of smoking deaths are attributable to lung cancer, throat cancer, and emphysema. Everyone knows that. But did you know that people who smoke one pack of cigarettes a day double their risk of heart attack? A full one-fifth of heart attack deaths are attributable to smoking. And women smokers open themselves up to heart attack risk *19 years* earlier than non-smoking women. Almost two decades! Smoking is one factor (diabetes is another) that negates the pre-menopausal protection against heart disease.

Cigarette smoke has chemicals that accelerate plaque formation. And smoking seems to change the environment of the artery, irritating it and putting it into defensive repair mode, meaning an increased likelihood of clot formation. It can interrupt your normal heart rhythm as well as raise your blood pressure. It can negatively affect your cholesterol level. It leads to heart disease in and of itself but it can also contribute dangerously to the other risk factors. If you tally it up, it works out like this: for every cigarette you smoke, you lose ten minutes of your life.

And the risk is greater for women than men. Studies are finding that the toxic chemicals in cigarette smoke are more lethal for women. Female smokers have an increased risk of heart disease compared to male smokers. Worse, we have a harder time quitting. With women, there seems to be more of a fixation on the actual *act* of smoking. Men respond better to nicotine patches or gum when

Shyla T. High, M.D.

trying to curb their addiction. Nicotine substitutions don't seem to work quite so well with women, who miss the tactile component of holding and smoking a cigarette.

It doesn't help that the cigarette companies spend a disproportionate amount of their advertising budgets targeting women. Teen girls in particular are wooed with messages of stylish sophistication. Smoking is made to look glamorous. Unfortunately, the insidious marketing efforts seem to be working. Nearly one in five of us take up the habit.

Obesity, Physical Inactivity, Diet

Close on the heels of smoking for modifiable heart disease factors is obesity. Obesity is a relatively new problem in the history of humanity. We've reached a point in our modernized, industrialized world where obesity has become more of a health risk than starvation! More than one-third of American adults are obese. The latest predictions are that by 2030, almost half of us will be obese. Obesity has become nothing less than an epidemic.

Obesity increases the risk of heart disease in and of itself, but, like smoking, it can contribute to the other risk factors as well, especially high blood pressure, cholesterol, and the chances of developing diabetes. What exactly does it mean to be obese? A lot of my patients think of the word as a sort of general term meaning overweight, or very overweight, but the term "obese" is actually tied to a specific measurement called the body mass index (BMI). The BMI measures body fat and takes into account weight and height. You can find a BMI table in the appendix. Find your BMI and see where you fall:

Body Mass Index

Under 18.5	Underweight
18.5 – 24.9	Normal
25 – 29.9	Overweight
30+	Obese

Not to complicate the matter, but there appears to be another important factor besides BMI, and that's the *distribution* of weight. Studies indicate that women with a higher distribution of weight around the belly (so-called "apple-shaped" women as opposed to "pear-shaped") have a higher risk of heart disease. And this seems to hold true even if the overall BMI is normal. Either way, excess weight, no matter where it ends up, should be addressed for good heart health.

Although genetics can be involved, there are two modifiable risk factors that, individually and together, have a big impact on whether a person will

Shyla T. High, M.D.

become obese: a person's level of physical activity and a person's diet. Lack of exercise and poor nutritional habits can lead to obesity, as well as lead to high blood pressure, high cholesterol, and the onset of diabetes. And of course each of those can lead directly to heart disease. We'll spend a little more time on physical activity and diet in the next chapter.

High Blood Pressure

High blood pressure is dangerous because it means the force of your blood as it's being pumped along your arteries and blood vessels is greater than it should be. The heart is being overworked. As a result, this can lead to congestive heart failure, arrhythmias, and a predisposition to heart attacks and strokes. High blood pressure also adds to the buildup of plaque in your arteries, requiring even greater force for the blood to be pumped through. High blood pressure, like heart disease itself, is another one of those conditions that are often thought of as male dominated. The truth, however, is that almost a third of U.S. women have high blood pressure and over the age of 55, more women than men have it.

90% of the time, high blood pressure comes with no underlying explanation. Called "essential hypertension," it just shows up, sometimes as we age. The other 10% of the time, high blood pressure can be traced either to medical reasons (like a thyroid or kidney condition), or to lifestyle factors (smoking, for example, or diet).

The measurement of blood pressure has two components, the systolic pressure, the pressure of the blood as the heart is beating; and diastolic pressure, the pressure between beats. (The pressure is measured in millimeters of mercury, or mm HG.)

Whether your blood pressure is considered normal, you have pre-hypertension (meaning you may be likely to develop high blood pressure), you have high blood pressure (Stage 1), or you have very high blood pressure (Stage 2), depends on where your measurement falls in the table below.

	Systolic (mm HG)	Diastolic (mm HG)
Normal	Less than 120	Less than 80
Pre-hypertension	120-139	80-89
STAGE 1 High Blood Pressure	140-159	90-99
STAGE 2 High Blood Pressure	160+	100+

The problem with high blood pressure is that many times it's asymptomatic. Absent taking a measurement on a regular basis, you'll have very little awareness that you have it, if any awareness at all. High blood pressure isn't called the silent killer for

Shyla T. High, M.D.

nothing. It typically doesn't announce its presence with pain or discomfort. It doesn't keep you up at night. It doesn't make you obviously tired or take away your appetite. If symptoms do occur, they're typically vague and subtle—fatigue, for example, or a headache or some other non-specific discomfort. A person can go years (and many do) without having any idea they have high blood pressure. And all of that time, this silent killer can be leading you to heart disease.

With high blood pressure, the key is to be proactive. Know what your blood pressure is. You don't have to wait to go to your doctor's office to find out. You can buy a blood pressure monitor in any drug store. They're inexpensive and a great investment in your heart health. Take your blood pressure regularly, keeping in mind that there are natural ebbs and flows. Expect some variability. For most people, their blood pressure is highest between 5:00 and 9:00 in the morning. So take it at different times and note any pattern of pre-hypertension or numbers that fall into the high ranges.

If you know you have high blood pressure and you're already on blood pressure medication, take your blood pressure before you take your medication, then take it again 12 hours later. Blood pressure medications are typically 24-hour drugs, working at their peak at 12 hours. That's the best point at which to assess the efficacy of your medication. There's typically no reason to check it any more than that unless circumstances warrant it. There's nothing wrong with a little diligence, of course, but if you find yourself becoming obsessed with your blood pressure, wanting to check it every 15 minutes, you might only succeed in creating stress for yourself that may end up contributing to the very thing you're trying to avoid!

Cholesterol

Cholesterol, like high blood pressure, is another silent killer. Know your cholesterol numbers, especially your LDL level. God gives every cell cholesterol, but a high **LDL** measurement (*low*-density lipoproteins, which I tell my patients to remember as "lousy" cholesterol) means you're at an increased risk of having fat accumulate along the walls of your arteries. If there's too much LDL, the arteries will take it up and it will build up along the artery walls as plaque.

But there's good cholesterol, too. A high **HDL** measurement (*high*-density lipoproteins, which I tell my patients to remember as "healthy" or "happy" cholesterol) means you have an abundance of a type of cholesterol that binds to the lousy (LDL) cholesterol and takes it to the liver to be excreted as stool.

The importance, however, of a high HDL level has been thrown into question with the most recent medical findings. Although people with high HDL levels seem to have less risk of heart attack, it's not really known what the nature of the relationship is. Raising your HDL level (through medication) might not help as much as once thought. Regardless, a low HDL level is considered something of a red flag and so it's important to know your HDL. Know your triglyceride level, too. Triglycerides are another form of fat, the high presence of which has been linked to atherosclerosis and, consequently, heart disease.

Everyone over the age of 20 ought to have their cholesterol levels tested at least once every five years, and women over the age of 45, more frequently. Here are the ranges, according to the latest guidelines from the American Heart Association[*]:

LDL Level (milligrams per deciliter)

Less than 100: Optimal

100-129: Above optimal

130-159: Borderline high

160-189: High

190+ : Very high

HDL Level (milligrams per deciliter)

Less than 60: Too low; major risk factor

60+ : Favorable; much less risk

Triglyceride Level (milligrams per deciliter)

Less than 150: Normal

150-199: Borderline high

200-499: High

500+ : Very high

Other tests exist, too. A lipoprotein particle count (lipoprotein NMR or Apo B [apolipoprotein B] profile), counts the actual particles that carry your cholesterol through the bloodstream and can be a valuable measurement of risk. Since 50% of heart attack victims have normal cholesterol numbers, it's important to consider more in-depth testing, like a lipoprotein particle count, if you're living with other high-risk factors for heart disease. The more information you can access about your heart disease risk, the better.

Diabetes

Diabetes is a danger all by itself. A serious risk from being overweight to obese, diabetes is a metabolic disorder where the body's cells fail to use insulin properly, a hormone that triggers otherwise healthy cells to take up glucose (sugar) from the blood so as to store it (in the form of glycogen) for when the body needs energy. When the cells don't

Shyla T. High, M.D.

do what they're supposed to do with glucose, the blood runs rampant with it and bad things can result. Diabetes can also come about as a result of a genetic predisposition and sometimes even from certain medications. Short-term problems can include hyperglycemia, which, if left acutely untreated, can lead to a coma (or worse). Long-term consequences can include kidney damage, blindness, peripheral vascular disease including strokes, and, of course, heart disease. Diabetes doubles the risk of heart disease for men, but increases it in women by three to five times!

Intertwined

By now, if you've noticed nothing else, you've noticed how intertwined all of these risk factors are. In fact, doctors have a term—metabolic syndrome—to describe a condition where a patient has at least three of these specific risk factors: high blood pressure, abnormal lipids (high Triglycerides, low HDL), elevated fasting glucose, and abdominal obesity measured as waist circumference. It's estimated that as much as 25% of the adult U.S. population suffers from metabolic syndrome. I'd use another term to describe this lethal combination: heart attack waiting to happen.

Metabolic Syndrome information:
http://tinyurl.com/AHA-MHS

Fortunately, the intertwining of these factors makes them easier to fight. Addressing one can have a favorable impact on the others. With a few, simple lifestyle changes, you can make a big difference overall.

Pulse Points

- Heart disease is when plaque builds up in the arteries of the heart causing a dangerous thickening of the artery walls.

- A heart attack is when a clot develops in an already-narrowed artery, thus preventing the flow of blood.

- Non-modifiable risk factors for heart disease are age and genetics.

- Modifiable risk factors include smoking, obesity, physical inactivity, blood pressure, cholesterol, and diabetes.

- One-fifth of heart attack deaths are attributable to smoking.

- Women smokers risk heart attacks *19 years* earlier than non-smoking women.

Shyla T. High, M.D.

- For every cigarette you smoke, you lose ten minutes of your life.

- By 2030, almost half of the adult U.S. population will be obese.

- A person can go years without having any idea they have high blood pressure—the silent killer.

- Know what your blood pressure is.

- Know your cholesterol numbers.

- Diabetes increases the risk of heart disease for women by three to five times.

- With a few, simple lifestyle changes, you can greatly reduce your risk of developing heart disease.

Shyla T. High, M.D.

CHAPTER THREE

Heal Thyself

Do-It-Yourself Heart Health

I find that a lot of my patients really don't know just how in control they are of their heart health. Of the modifiable risk factors we discussed in the last chapter, the top three—smoking, obesity, and physical inactivity—are risk factors you can address yourself. Before making even one trip to your doctor's office or pharmacy, you can positively affect your heart health significantly just by finding a way to reduce these three factors.

The news gets even better when you stop to consider that the top three factors often times have an effect on the other three. The risks from high blood pressure, high cholesterol, and the threat of diabetes can frequently be lessened considerably if you reduce your risks from smoking, obesity, and physical inactivity.

Becoming Smoke-Free

If you're a smoker, and you do nothing else to reduce your risk of heart disease, stop smoking. It's really that simple. Smoking is by far the riskiest of all the risk factors. And dropping the habit produces very quick results. Immediately the environment of your arteries changes. They become healthier. Quitting won't necessarily reverse the plaque buildup, but it will calm down the irritated arteries, reducing the chance of clot formation. Within two days, your chances of having a heart attack become reduced. After one year, those chances are cut in half.

If you smoke, find a way to stop. If it's too overwhelming to think about, remember that it needn't be all at once. Take baby steps; cut back and then cut back again. Keep cutting. You can do it. I'm convinced that a pack-a-day smoker smokes 20 cigarettes a day for no other reason than that's how many are in a pack. If a pack had 18 cigarettes, you'd smoke 18. If it had 15, you'd smoke 15. Set a realistic timeline for quitting and keep reducing the number of cigarettes you smoke each day until that number is zero.

Eating for Heart Health

I'm often asked by patients to recommend a good diet, but I'm not too keen on doing so because

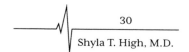

I don't believe in dietary quick fixes. There are diets available that will allow you to drop fifty pounds in no time. But that doesn't mean they're healthy. Or even effective in the long run. Once you drop the weight, the weight typically comes back. Need some proof? A third of Americans report being on a diet at any given time and yet we keep getting fatter. Something obviously isn't working.

What's required to lose weight and to subsequently *maintain* a healthy weight, is not a diet, but a change in eating habits, a change in lifestyle. A long-term approach to eating and not a quick fix.

Generally-speaking, most women should eat around 2,000 calories per day, though that number can vary depending on your level of physical activity. If you're exercising regularly and successfully burning off calories, you can afford a higher caloric intake than a sedentary person. Regardless of the total calories, no more than a fourth of them (500 if your daily caloric intake is 2,000) should come from fat.

As important as the quantity of food is the quality. Here are some recommendations from the American Heart Association* for heart-healthy eating:

• Fruits and vegetables: At least 4.5 cups a day;

• Fish (preferably oily fish): At least two 3.5-ounce servings a week;

- Fiber-rich whole grains: At least three 1-ounce-equivalent servings a day;

- Sodium: Less than 1,500 mg a day;

- Sugar-sweetened beverages: No more than 450 calories (36 ounces) a week.

Other dietary considerations from the American Heart Association:

- Nuts, legumes and seeds: At least 4 servings a week;

- Processed meats: No more than 2 servings a week;

- Saturated fat: Less than 7% of total energy intake.

*Reprinted with Permission, www.heart.org. ©2012 American Heart Association, Inc.

Within these simple guidelines, you can be amazingly creative with your meals. All it takes is some imagination, or, at the least, an imaginative cookbook. Dozens of heart-healthy recipe books are available.

For the most part, it's a case of moderation in your diet. You don't have to spend your time in diet

Shyla T. High, M.D.

jail. You can eat well, and you can eat decent portions, and you can still maintain (or lose) weight. Pay attention to your caloric intake, and focus on heart-healthy foods. It's easy.

To make it even easier, I tell my patients they can take one day off a week. I know from experience with my patients that deprivation often leads to frustration which often leads to abandoning even the most relaxed diet. This is why starvation diets never work. Go ahead and treat yourself one day of the week to those foods you keep away from the rest of the week but still might have the occasional craving for. It'll satisfy your hunger and make the rest of the week just that much easier.

Once you learn to successfully moderate your diet, you'll gain motivation by seeing the results—dropped pounds, more attractive figure, more energy. But the significance of a healthy diet is such that physiological benefits show up even faster than you can spot them. Even five pounds can have a huge impact on your heart health. So just because you may not be losing weight at the rate you'd like, or aren't yet seeing any visible results, your heart can tell the difference. Just like smoking, your task needn't be overwhelming. A little change for the positive, a baby-step forward with the loss of just a few pounds, helps a great deal. Getting started is the key. Then, keep at it.

Get Yourself Moving

Like smoking and diet, adding physical activity into your life doesn't need to be overwhelming either. Being physically active doesn't mean you need a daily two-hour workout at your local fitness club. You don't even have to call it "exercise." Just get yourself out of your chair and do something that increases your heart and lung activity. You'll increase your circulation and lower your blood pressure. All of this can happen with a 30-minute brisk walk every day.

Physical activity burns calories, too. So, coupled with a healthy diet of moderation, you'll lose fat. 180 calories can be burned during that 30-minute walk. Twice as many if you make the walk an hour. Gardening, bicycling, dancing—you can burn as much doing any of these. You can burn more than 600 calories an hour if you jog or swim. Find a physical activity you like to do and do it.

Little by Little

The fact is, fighting the risk factors of smoking, obesity, and physical inactivity can—individually, and especially collectively—have a positive effect on your heart health. And small changes in all of them can have a big impact. You don't have to stop smoking cold turkey today, lose 100 pounds by next week, and start running marathons by next month. But little by little, you can make a huge difference in your health. Stick with it. Set goals and timetables. Make the goals and timetables realistic, but don't be afraid to push yourself. The stakes are high. No less than life and death.

And, as mentioned, taking it upon yourself to reduce your risk of heart disease from these three factors can work towards reducing your risk from the other three—high blood pressure, high cholesterol, and diabetes. I've had patients able to wean themselves off of their high blood pressure medication just by diet alone. But the main thing to remember is this: it's much easier to prevent heart disease than to correct it.

Start now.

Pulse Points

♥ *You* are in control of your heart health.

♥ Reducing and/or eliminating your risk of heart disease from smoking, obesity, and physical inactivity is something you don't even need a doctor for.

♥ If you're a smoker, your top health priority is easy to choose: stop smoking.

- An effective diet is one you can live with for the rest of your life, not a quick fix that's impossible to maintain.

- Pay attention to your caloric intake and focus on heart-healthy foods.

- Consistent physical activity (a brisk walk) for even 30 minutes makes a difference.

- Small changes can add up. You don't have to accomplish everything at once. But getting started on the road to preventing heart disease is much, much easier than dealing with actual heart disease.

Shyla T. High, M.D.

CHAPTER FOUR

Symptoms and Tests

Am I Having a Heart Attack?

A heart attack, technically referred to as a myocardial infarction (M.I.), is a complete blockage of a coronary artery. Symptoms can take several forms. As we discussed earlier, it's not always chest pains one feels, and this is especially so in women. Symptoms leading up to a heart attack can include shortness of breath or extreme fatigue, sweating, and dizziness. But the classic symptom remains the feeling, not so much of pain actually, but of intense pressure in the chest. It's not like a shooting pain or a pain like a headache pain or when you stub your toe. Patients who have had heart attacks often report that they felt as though an elephant was sitting on their chest. It's a tightness. Some women report that it feels as though their bra is *way* too snug.

Of course chest pain can also result from partial blockage. This pain can typically be categorized as either stable or unstable angina. Stable angina, as the name implies, is characterized by some consistency in how you experience it. You might feel it regularly or even predictably whenever you exert yourself to a certain extent. It probably doesn't last very long and goes away when you rest. Unstable angina, on the other hand, is more unexpected. Sudden pain that might not even require exertion before it starts, or pain that doesn't go away when you rest. It might, in fact, be a signal of a heart attack.

Of course there are other reasons besides a heart attack or angina that might cause one to feel chest pain or tightness. Indigestion is a common one. What makes cardiac pain unique, however, is the physical exertion or situational stress that normally precedes it. If your arteries are blocked, there's going to be a certain level of heart rate that's going to put such a demand on your heart that your arteries, built up with plaque, aren't going to be able to accommodate the necessary blood flow. And when you hit that heart rate, the chest discomfort begins—the feeling of tightness and pressure.

Other symptoms might occur as well. Sweating and nausea, for example. Sweating rarely accompanies indigestion. So if physical exertion has led to chest pains that are accompanied by sweating, you don't need to be a cardiologist to suspect a heart attack.

In addition to chest pains (which, remember, might *not* be present), and in addition to sweating, nausea, fatigue, dizziness, and shortness of breath, other symptoms might include a radiating pain in the upper body, typically on the left side, or pain in the neck or jaw. Of course these symptoms might indicate other conditions and we'll talk about them later. The point is, there's never a reason to take a chance. If you suspect you or someone you're with is having a heart attack, *call 911!* Immediately. With the heart, time is muscle. The longer you wait, the more damage will be done.

Stress Tests

If there's not 100% blockage, that is to say that if an actual heart attack isn't taking place or has been ruled out by medically-established criteria (or if the patient isn't experiencing *un*stable angina), but symptoms are present that *may* indicate some level of blockage, then there's a test available that can confirm or disconfirm that indication: the exercise stress test. This test replicates the kind of exertion that might cause chest pain from too much demand being put on a heart whose arteries are clogged with plaque.

Typically the test employs the use of a treadmill, (although a stationary bike can also be used). We start with a 10% grade and have the patient walk at 2.5 miles-per-hour for three minutes. Then we bump the grade up at every three-minute interval. (For the bike test, more resistance is added every three minutes making it increasingly harder to pedal.) What we're trying to do is elevate the patient's heart rate to a protocol-established target rate of 85% of the patient's maximum rate (as determined by age). If we can do that without reproducing the symptoms the patient initially complained about, or have other classic heart disease symptoms appear, the test is considered negative from a symptom standpoint and lends a favorable overall prognosis. On the other hand, having to stop the test due to chest pain or pressure automatically qualifies as a positive test result.

A negative stress test means not only getting to your target rate with no chest discomfort, but also having no problems show up on the accompanying electrocardiogram. While the patient is taking the test, we monitor the heart's electrical activity using an electrocardiogram or EKG. An EKG provides us with a printout of the heart's activity as a series of waves.

Shyla T. High, M.D.

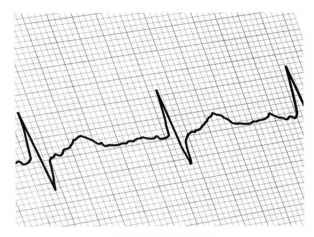

ILLUSTRATION 2. **EKG**

We'll do an EKG before the patient gets on the treadmill and then during, comparing the results to look for abnormalities. These abnormalities may show up with or without chest pain. And of course we look for other symptoms, too, like extreme shortness of breath or marked fatigue. These symptoms, while the heart is under stress, tell us we may have a problem.

The very latest research informs us that with asymptomatic patients, routine EKGs are unnecessary. But if somewhere along the line your doctor has, for whatever reason, performed an EKG on you, that information might be valuable. But only in so far as it relates to a future EKG. A single EKG is a snapshot in time, a graph of your heart's electrical activity on a certain day. It's most useful as a baseline standard of comparison. It's the changes we're interested in from one EKG to the next. You'll hear about someone having a heart attack whose EKG was perfectly normal six months ago. But that was six months ago. An EKG performed a week ago might have indicated a significant change from the one performed six months ago, and it's that change, along with other symptoms, that might have clued us in on any impending danger.

Changes in EKGs are an important bellwether. Abnormalities, especially in post-menopausal women, have been determined to be a means by which to predict heart attacks, heart disease, or stroke all by themselves; that is to say even without any other symptoms present or confirming tests. In a recent study detailed in the *Journal of the American Medical Association* (March, 2007, Dr. Pablo Denes), it was found that EKG abnormalities were associated with three times the risk of coronary heart disease in postmenopausal women.

In some cases I may elect to use a *nuclear* stress test. Fortunately, this isn't as frightening as it sounds. With a nuclear stress test a chemical, called a radio-tracer, is injected into the patient before she gets on the treadmill. This material emits rays from the heart from which a special camera can produce an image. We look at an image before exertion, and another

Shyla T. High, M.D.

one after. Comparing the two images, we can spot areas of low blood flow, areas that have some blockage, in other words. In other cases, I might use an echocardiogram test. This is essentially a sonogram for the heart. Using sound waves, the test produces, like the nuclear test, images of the heart before and after the treadmill exercise.

Sometimes a patient isn't a good candidate for the treadmill or stationary bike. Maybe the patient's resting EKG is already showing signs of an abnormality. Maybe it would be too risky to put her on the treadmill. Or maybe the patient is obese, or has bad knees, or there's some other reason she can't get on the treadmill. In those cases, we can chemically replicate stress. We can inject the patient with a medication that increases blood flow to the heart without having the patient have to exert herself physically.

The type of stress test you might undergo will depend on a number of factors and your primary care physician or cardiologist is the best person to determine just what test is right for you given your specific circumstances. There is no one-size-fits-all test. If I have a real strong suspicion of heart disease, I might go with a nuclear test or echocardiogram, tests that are a bit more sensitive than the EKG. I like the echocardiogram, but in some instances (women with very large breasts, for example) it's not practical. Your level of conditioning or resting EKG might determine whether I replicate exertion chemically, rather than put you on the treadmill.

In other words, testing, just like treatment, is best undertaken with a customized approach. Trust your doctor to proceed in the best way for you. One way to ensure this is to be honest with your doctor. It's important that you and your doctor have the kind of relationship where you can be completely open about your health. Truthfully, about 85% of a heart disease diagnosis comes from the patient's own words! It's the patient's history right from the patient's mouth that provides the most important element of heart disease assessment. Probably 10% is a physical examination. That leaves 5% for testing. As important as testing is, its major purpose is to confirm existing suspicions. And without the suspicions, the testing might not take place. Talk to your doctor. If your doctor can't read your mind, so he or she can't read your heart.

Screening for Heart Disease

Where the stress test is used to assess heart disease symptoms to confirm whether or not heart disease is present, there are other tests available that look for plaque buildup, screening for heart disease even if there are no symptoms. One such screening

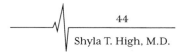

Shyla T. High, M.D.

method is the CT scan (computerized tomographic scan). A CT scan (sometimes called a CAT scan) uses special x-ray equipment to produce cross-sectional images of the inside of the body. A *cardio* CT scan focuses, as you may expect, on the heart and produces images that reveal coronary calcium—calcified plaque buildup. The extent is graded as a "calcium score" and gives the doctor evidence as to the degree of plaque buildup.

The cardio CT scan can be combined with the injection of a dye in a screening test called a CT angiography (or CTA test). The CTA test provides more detailed imagery of the arteries.

Here's the thing about tests that screen for heart disease, as opposed to tests that assess existing symptoms (i.e., stress tests). Most of the time the approach is the same whether you have 10% blockage or 60% blockage. The preventive measures we discussed in the last chapter—if taken seriously and carried out diligently—represent your best chance at reversing your plaque buildup. My concern is when a patient's blockage becomes severe enough to produce symptoms. That, of course, warrants a stress test to confirm or disconfirm the existence of heart disease. The fact is, learning that a patient has some degree of plaque buildup, or no plaque buildup at all, isn't really going to alter my advice for living a healthy life, a smoke-free life in which you eat well and keep physically active. So, is it really helpful to ascertain the precise level of plaque buildup? If your doctor recommends a screening test, maybe he or she has a good reason for doing so. From my professional perspective: 1) don't hesitate to act upon any symptoms that may indicate heart trouble, and, better still, 2) live a lifestyle that'll keep those symptoms from ever appearing in the first place. Knowing the exact amount of plaque buildup might satisfy your (or your doctor's) curiosity, but it typically won't change these two approaches to heart-healthy living.

Importance

The importance of paying attention to your body and noting symptoms of potential heart disease cannot be overemphasized. Serious symptoms need to be dealt with immediately, via a 911 phone call. Serious or not-so-serious, your doctor needs to be informed so that he or she can arrange, if appropriate, the right test for you to determine if heart disease is a real and present threat.

Remember—more women than men die within one year of having a heart attack. And of the survivors, more women than men will develop congestive heart failure within five years and will have more complications resulting from bypass surgeries. This underscores the importance for

Shyla T. High, M.D.

women especially to detect potential heart disease upfront, *before* it ends up resulting in a heart attack.

Pulse Points

+ It's not always chest pain you feel when you're having a heart attack. But if it is, it's typically a tightening in the chest or a feeling of extreme pressure.

+ Chest pain related to a heart event results from physical exertion; the arteries cannot handle the increased demand for blood flow.

+ If you suspect a heart attack—call 911 immediately. Time is muscle.

+ A stress test (usually a treadmill or stationary bike) will replicate the conditions that might cause chest pain, thus confirming or disconfirming heart disease.

+ An EKG is a printout of your heart's activity and is at its most valuable when compared to previous EKGs.

+ Nuclear stress tests and echocardiograms are tests that increase the accuracy of detecting significant blockage.

- A good, open working relationship with your doctor or cardiologist is the best way to make certain you're going to get the testing and treatment that's best for you.

- Screening for plaque with tests such as the CT scan or CTA can reveal levels of plaque, but, absent symptomatic blockage, preventive measures including lifestyle changes will be the recommended course of treatment regardless of level.

- Detecting heart disease up front—before a heart attack—is always important, but even more so for women.

Shyla T. High, M.D.

CHAPTER FIVE

So if it's Not a Heart Attack, What is It?

Might be the Heart. Might not be the Heart.

It's no surprise that a heart attack can be a source of chest pain. But there are a few other cardiac reasons that might cause chest pain, too. We've already discussed angina. Additionally, there are aortic dissection, pericarditis, coronary spasms, and heart palpitations, all of which may produce some degree of chest pain. And there are a lot of non-cardiac reasons, too. Let's rule out the cardiac ones first.

Cardiac Chest Pain

Of all the cardiac related causes of chest pain, the scariest may be **aortic dissection**. This might be even more frightening than a heart attack. Aortic dissection is a tear that takes place in the lining of the aorta wall. If it tears completely open, a victim can literally bleed to death internally, and quickly. Half the victims die before they even reach a hospital. If caught in time it can be treated surgically. Often it's diagnosed with an M.R.I. Probably the most famous recent case of aortic dissection is the case of actor John Ritter. Ritter's condition was ultimately determined to be from an undiagnosed congenital defect, but the most common cause is a lifetime of hypertension. Fortunately, aortic dissection is rather rare, occurring in only about 1 of every 5,000 people, and is most common in men between the ages of 50-70.

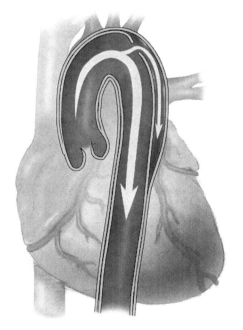

ILLUSTRATION 3. **AORTIC DISSECTION**

Shyla T. High, M.D.

More common, but much less worrisome, is **pericarditis**. Pericarditis is an inflammation of the pericardium, the sac that surrounds your heart. Typically its cause is viral but it can be caused by a bacterial infection as well. It can be thought of as similar to pleurisy, which is an inflammation of the lining surrounding the lungs. Chest pain is a common symptom but it's a different kind of pain than the chest pain associated with a heart attack. It's more of a sharp pain, as opposed to a pressure or crushing kind of pain. And it comes about with no regard to level of physical exertion. It's more acute in different positions, too, sometimes more obvious when you take a deep breath. Though pericarditis can become a very serious condition, for the most part it's fairly treatable with medication. Mild cases might even clear up on their own.

A **coronary artery spasm** is a contraction of the artery wall muscles. It's a muscle spasm, in other words. But the sudden contraction can constrict the artery and interfere, even halt, the flow of blood. Spasms are more common in people with heart disease but they can also be triggered by extreme stress and often by chemical stimulants. It's a danger for cocaine users and for those who abuse amphetamines. A coronary artery spasm, though not a heart attack, can lead to a heart attack if the artery becomes completely restricted. In that case, the end result isn't any different than if the artery becomes completely clogged by plaque: the flow of blood stops and the heart muscle begins to die.

At one time or another, almost everyone experiences **heart palpitations**. Rapid or skipped heartbeats can be caused by stress, too much caffeine, nicotine, certain medications, and strong physical exertion. Sometimes hormonal changes can cause heart palpitations—changes due to pregnancy or menopause, or even menstruation. The fluttering feeling of palpitations, or the feeling of a missed heart beat can sometimes feel like chest pressure or discomfort. Palpitations are rarely serious. They're not specific to blockage and more or less represent, instead, a very brief electrical problem. Such a problem in the setting of a structurally normal heart is typically benign.

Non-Cardiac Chest Pain

Here's the good news. 80% of chest pain is not heart-related. But if it's not heart-related, what else could your chest pain be? Non-cardiac chest discomfort breaks down into four major causes. **Musculoskeletal** is the most common. This kind of pain might be represented by stress and strain of cartilage or ribs. Costochondritis is a condition where the cartilage that connects a rib to the breastbone becomes inflamed, typically caused by injury or maybe physical strain. But it can also be caused by an infection and it's sometimes seen in people with arthritis, too. Women are more prone to costochondritis than men. Because of its location, right at the breastbone, it can feel like the kind of pain you might expect during a heart attack. But, like pericarditis, and unlike heart attack pain, the severity of the pain might be dependent on one's physical positioning. Twisting and turning a certain way might aggravate it. Conversely, remaining still might cause the pain to subside. If the pain can be reproduced by certain movements, you're probably experiencing some form of musculoskeletal problem. In time, musculoskeletal pain like costochondritis normally goes away on its own by allowing the area in question to heal by limiting the type of movement that's aggravating it. Your doctor might also prescribe pain medication or anti-inflammatory drugs and, in the case of an infection, an antibiotic.

A second non-cardiac cause of chest discomfort is **gastrointestinal**. Acid reflux or its more serious form, Gastroesophageal reflux disease (GERD), is the prime example. There's a reason they call it heartburn. Other intestinal issues that might result in chest pain would include pancreatitis, ulcers, and gall bladder problems. These may come with associated symptoms like bloating or belching, symptoms that aren't typically present with cardiac events. A doctor's diagnosis is important in nailing down the cause so that the right treatment can be offered. Simple reflux can often be prevented by the avoidance of certain foods. More serious gastrointestinal cases might require more involved treatment. Either way, if gastrointestinal issues are suspected with your chest pain, it's pretty easy for your doctor to rule out a cardiac cause.

Respiratory problems can also create chest pain. Pleurisy, which we mentioned before, an inflammation of the lining that surrounds the lungs, can produce a constricting feeling in the chest. So can a collapsed lung, as you might imagine, although collapsed lungs are rare, especially without some kind of physical trauma (a car accident, for instance). Pleurisy can often be treated with antibiotics if the cause is from an infection. There are other causes, too, which your doctor will be able to determine. I see it from time to time as a post-operative complication of heart surgery.

The most serious respiratory problem is a pulmonary embolism. This is a blockage of an artery, or arteries, in your lungs, typically caused by a blood clot that was formed elsewhere in the body and traveled into the lungs. The blockage can literally starve the lungs of air and can become life-threatening in a hurry. Symptoms are similar to those of a heart

Shyla T. High, M.D.

attack—chest pain and shortness of breath. A cough might also be present. Frequently the clots are formed in the legs (known as deep vein thrombosis or DVT) and often they are caused by lengthy stretches of immobility. A fairly recent instance was the fatal case of NBC news correspondent David Bloom, embedded with a U.S. infantry division in Iraq in 2003. From remaining stationary for hours in a tank, he developed a DVT which subsequently traveled into his lungs. The threat of a pulmonary embolism is why travelers flying, driving, or riding for long distances are encouraged to get up and stretch their legs every hour or so.

The final cause of non-cardiac chest pain is **psychological** in nature. This would include chest pain from anxiety, stress, or outright panic attacks. Why stress sometimes leads to pain in the chest isn't really well understood. But it's easy to confuse it with a cardiac event since the adrenaline present in a period of great stress often creates a pounding or rapid heartbeat. And then of course the anxiety of a perceived heart attack only adds to the stress which in turn adds to the chest pain! Interestingly, panic disorders that create chest pain are most common in women under 30.

Chest discomfort from psychological reasons is not all that uncommon and the pain normally subsides when the stress or anxiety eventually abates.

Often, long term treatment involves stress management and the development of coping mechanisms to better handle anxiety or head off a potential panic attack.

Treatment

Treatment for chest pain depends on determining the cause. Sometimes that requires a multipronged approach. Maybe the cause is determined in the emergency room, or maybe by your primary care physician, or maybe by a specialist that your primary care physician sends you to. Always, the first priority is ruling out a real cardiac threat, whether it's a heart attack, aortic dissection, or, perhaps, a pulmonary embolism. Once the life-threatening causes are dealt with, then the less threatening, and more common, causes can be addressed. As always, making a guess yourself can be dangerous. If you're experiencing chest pains, call 911.

Shyla T. High, M.D.

Pulse Points

- Chest pain doesn't necessarily mean heart attack, although it can be cardiac related.

- Sources of cardiac chest pain include aortic dissection, pericarditis, coronary artery spasm, or heart palpitations.

- Source of non-cardiac chest pain include musculoskeletal, gastrointestinal, respiratory, and psychological.

- Treatment depends on the source and a definitive diagnosis might require a multipronged approach.

- Don't guess! If you're having serious heart discomfort, call 911.

CHAPTER SIX

So You're Having a Heart Attack

Your Heart Attack Action Plan

If you think you or someone you're with is having a heart attack, you need to take action immediately, beginning with a phone call to 911. And only 911. Many times valuable minutes are lost with calls to a primary care physician. If you're experiencing chest pains, or other heart attack symptoms, your doctor is only going to tell you to hang up and dial 911 anyway. And the best chance of survival with minimum heart damage is a trip to the emergency room *via ambulance*. Do not attempt to drive yourself to the hospital. The most serious early heart attack complication is a rhythm abnormality and the paramedics who respond to the 911 call have the means, with the use of a defibrillator, to shock the heart back into rhythm. They can also give you oxygen and medication. Their quick work can be lifesaving. Studies have shown that people who arrive at the hospital in an ambulance get treated faster than those who drive themselves, and many times the treatment starts in the ambulance itself. Remember that with a heart attack, time is muscle. The longer treatment is delayed, the more heart damage is done. And the greater risk of loss of life.

While you're waiting for the paramedics, chew a 325 mg. aspirin. Aspirin inhibits the formation of platelets in the blood system, cells that help the blood clot. Reducing platelet formation can help reduce the clotting that is occurring in the heart and causing the heart attack. But speed is of the essence. Chewing the aspirin, rather than swallowing it, is the quickest way to get it into the bloodstream. Of course if you've had heart related issues and your doctor has prescribed nitroglycerin tablets, take one of those.

Make sure you have a list handy of all the medications you're taking and what, if anything, you're allergic to. Since one never knows when, or where, one's going to have a heart attack, this is a list you should keep on your person at all times.

If you're with someone having a heart attack and the person's heart has stopped and/or the person is not breathing, you'll need to employ cardiopulmonary resuscitation. If you're reading this book and you're not familiar with CPR,

Shyla T. High, M.D.

visit the American Heart Association's website (www.heart.org) for instructional information. Let's hope you'll never need it, but your knowledge of CPR just might save a life someday.

At the Hospital

The emergency personnel who respond to the 911 call will take you to the nearest hospital for evaluation. A heart attack will be confirmed (or disconfirmed) by an EKG or possibly by a cardiac enzyme test. When heart muscle dies, certain enzymes are released into the bloodstream and a simple enzyme blood test can reveal whether or not a heart attack has taken place. A heart attack might also be confirmed in a doctor's mind simply by the presence of the classic heart attack symptoms.

Once confirmed, one of two things will happen. You may be treated with thrombolytics. These "clot busting" drugs are introduced intravenously and dissolve clots, thus restoring proper blood flow to the heart. Or, you may be recommended for an invasive procedure such as balloon angioplasty and/or a stent. The decision will depend on the doctor and perhaps the facility. If angioplasty capabilities aren't present and the doctor calls for angioplasty, you may need to be transferred elsewhere. Not all emergency facilities have angioplasty capabilities but all have clot busting medications. Notwithstanding the type of treatment available, the bottom line is that if you're having a heart attack, the best facility for you is the *nearest* one.

The Angiogram

The treatment of a heart attack will most frequently lead to an angiogram, also known as cardiac catheterization, often a prelude to angio-plasty and/or stenting, and a procedure that allows the doctor to pinpoint the blockage. But an angiogram might be ordered for other situations as well, such as:

• Unstable angina, also referred to as acute coronary syndrome (ACS). This might include worrisome symptoms or non-specific EKG changes;

• New onset angina, which is angina that's come on very recently in an otherwise healthy individual;

• Abnormal stress test results that would suggest the presence of heart disease;

• The presence of symptoms that are limiting one's functional capacity;

• The presence of symptoms in high-risk individ-uals, such as smokers or diabetics.

In an angiogram, a short plastic sheath is inserted into an artery, typically in the groin area. A catheter—a long, thin, flexible plastic tube—is inserted into the sheath and then threaded through the artery to your heart. A local anesthetic is used at the point of entry, and typically a mild sedative is

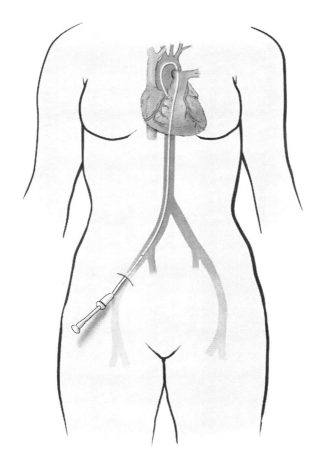

ILLUSTRATION 4. **ANGIOGRAM**

administered as well. After the catheter is in place, a special dye is injected into the catheter and with the help of an x-ray machine, angiographic images are taken that allow identification of the presence, or absence, of blockage. More importantly, the images tell the doctor precisely where the blockage is taking place.

If the angiogram is negative for heart disease severe enough to warrant a more immediate and invasive treatment (such as a stent as we'll discuss), then after a short period of recovery you can normally go home the same day. Since tests are performed beforehand that are pretty good indicators of significant heart disease (an EKG, for example, or a cardiac enzyme test), it's fairly likely that the angiogram will be positive. And that takes us to the next step.

Angioplasty and Stents

Angioplasty is the use of a tiny balloon, sent through the same catheter that's used to perform the angiogram, to open up the clogged vessel or vessels. Up until the early 1990s, that's all that was used. Since then, balloon angioplasty has been typically followed up with the stent—a tiny mesh tube that's inserted into the clogged vessel to act as a sort of scaffolding, keeping the vessel open.

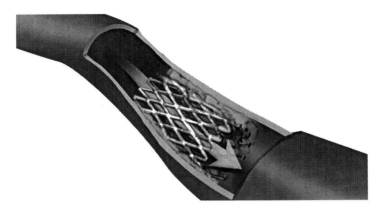

ILLUSTRATION 5. **STENT**

The stent is left in place permanently and a certain period of time is required to make certain it becomes properly incorporated into the vessel wall. Sometimes the stents are coated with medication to help keep scar tissue from developing around the stent and causing the vessel to narrow. Additionally, your doctor will most likely prescribe two aspirin-type products (Plavix, for example) for the same basic reason that you should chew an aspirin if you suspect you're having a heart attack: to keep platelets from forming and causing additional clotting. Your doctor will determine how long you'll need to take them. It might be a year or more. If there are other potential blockage issues besides the one that caused the heart attack, you might need to take them indefinitely.

If there are places of partial blockage that show up in the angiogram, your doctor will probably advise they be treated the same way in which you would treat general heart disease—with the same preventative measures outlined in Chapter Three, i.e. quit smoking, maintain a proper diet, stay physically active. If, however, there are other major points of blockage, your doctor may employ more than one stent. And in cases where there is acute heart disease or blockage is apparent in multiple places, you doctor may elect to go with bypass surgery.

Bypass Surgery

In bypass surgery, either an artery taken from the chest wall or a healthy vein typically taken from the leg is used to re-route the blood flow, bypassing a blocked or narrowed heart vessel. It becomes a frontage road of sorts, detouring highway traffic around a congested traffic tie-up, then back to the highway again. With the increasing use of stents, most people don't require bypass surgery, but it's still very common. And very effective in cases where stents might be inappropriate (with multiple blockages, as mentioned, or often in the case with diabetics who seem to respond better to bypass surgery than stents).

Shyla T. High, M.D.

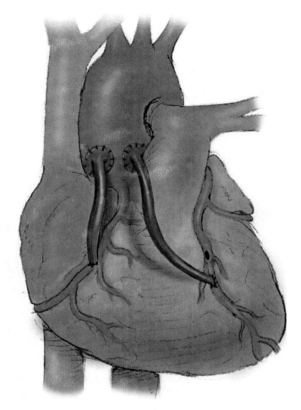

ILLUSTRATION 6. **BYPASS**

In rare cases, bypass surgery is done in an emergency situation such as during a heart attack. For the most part, though, it's done when the patient is stable and the doctor has determined that it's the best course of action given the condition of the patient's heart, normally within days of a heart attack.

The Difference with Women

We discussed earlier in the book the risks with women in particular of heart disease. Often with women a heart attack isn't properly diagnosed or isn't diagnosed in a timely enough manner. As you might expect, this has consequences for the effectiveness of the treatments we've covered in this chapter.

An interesting (and sobering) study that was outlined in the *New England Journal of Medicine* used actors to describe to doctors identical symptoms of heart attack pain.[2] What the study found was that the sex (as well as the race) of the actors played an influential part in the decisions those doctors made regarding treatment. This confirmed earlier studies that found basically the same thing: women are less likely than men to undergo potentially life-saving treatments like angiography. And this explains why emergency bypass surgery is more common with women than men; the symptoms are ignored until emergency bypass surgery becomes the only option left.

I've seen it myself. I had a patient come to me having been sent home from the emergency room not once, but twice. She'd had a heart attack that

---

[2] Schulman, K.A., Berlin, J.A., Harless, W., et al, "The Effect of Race and Sex on Physicians' Recommendations for Cardiac Catheterization", *New England Journal of Medicine*, 25 Feb., 1999; 340[8]:618-626.

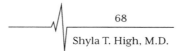

the E.R. staff missed. Fortunately, we were able to ultimately relieve her problems with stenting, but the outcome could have just as easily been tragic. Hopefully, as the medical world becomes more and more aware of today's increased risk of heart disease in women, these kinds of cases will become few and far between, if not altogether eliminated.

An Ounce of Prevention...

Not surprisingly, your best chance of survival is not to have a heart attack in the first place. Prevention is always the best treatment. And it's important to understand that clot busting drugs, angioplasty, stents, and bypass surgeries are not *cures* for heart disease. They are treatments after the fact. If you've had a heart attack, you can have one again. Your very life depends on preventing the conditions that caused the heart attack in the first place. Long-term success depends on lifestyle changes and healthy heart habits.

Pulse Points

- If you're having a heart attack, call 911 for an ambulance and chew (don't swallow) a 325 mg. aspirin.

- At the hospital, expect clot busting drugs and/or angiography.

- An angiogram will confirm the existence of blockage and show where exactly it is.

- Balloon angiography will open the blocked vessel and often serve as a prelude to stenting.

- Bypass surgery will be used in cases where stenting is inappropriate or would otherwise prove ineffective.

- The best heart attack treatment is not to have a heart attack in the first place!

Shyla T. High, M.D.

To Take or Not to Take: The Skinny on Meds

Primary, Secondary, What's the Difference?

With cardiovascular disease, doctors like to talk in terms of primary prevention and secondary prevention. Primary prevention describes the measures taken by people who haven't had heart attacks or perhaps have no real signs of heart disease, but remain at risk—people with high blood pressure, for example, or with high cholesterol. Secondary prevention describes the measures taken by people who have actually been diagnosed with heart disease. But here's what I think: in real, practical terms, there's not a whole lot of difference. Someone who's at high risk is a single blood clot away from going from primary to secondary prevention. The difference, but for treatment with a few select medications (statins, for instance), is largely semantic. So, primary or secondary, let's take a look at some of the medications your doctor might recommend for you and why.

Medication for Hypertension

In Chapter Two we discussed high blood pressure. If you'll recall, almost a third of American women have high blood pressure and over the age of 55, more women than men have it. Worse, essential hypertension is a silent killer, rarely announcing its presence with noticeable symptoms. The good news is that, with medication, high blood pressure is easy to get under control. What's unfortunate, even tragic, is that an estimated 70% of adults *don't* have their blood pressure under control, either because they don't know they have it or they know and ignore it. But with today's medications, there's absolutely no reason for you to have to live with suboptimal control of your high blood pressure.

If you have hypertension and your doctor advises treating it with medication, the type of medication will depend on several factors. As we'll soon see, there are several classes of medications available. Your doctor might prescribe just one, or he or she might prescribe a combination. Taken into consideration will be factors such as whether you have stage 1 or stage 2 high blood pressure (see Chapter Two), potential side effects of the medication, and whether you are being treated for other conditions. Your doctor will tailor the approach, in other words, to your specific circumstances. In the end, the value of any given approach will be measured by how it works towards the ultimate goal: lowering your blood pressure.

Let's talk about the various classes of blood pressure medications.

1. **Diuretics**. These so-called "water pills" are often used in combination with other high blood pressure meds. Their purpose is to help the kidneys rid the body of sodium, increasing the excretion of salt and water, and thereby decreasing the volume of blood that your heart has to pump through your veins. They're inexpensive and have other uses as well, such as for generalized swelling and congestive heart failure. Frequent urination is a common side effect of diuretics and they also have a tendency to deplete the body of potassium which can sometimes cause muscle cramping.

2. **ACE inhibitors**. Angiotensin converting enzymes are components of the blood pressure regulating system. Inhibiting them decreases the tension of your blood vessels. ACE inhibitors are

used for other diseases, too, like congestive heart failure, and they come with few side effects, the most common being a dry cough. But you'll want to call your doctor if you experience a swelling in the face, eyes, lips, or tongue.

3. **Beta blockers**. Beta blockers prevent certain neurotransmitters from attaching themselves to cell structures (called beta receptors) and stimulating the heart. Blocking those transmitters slows down the heart rate and causes the blood pressure to fall. Beta blockers also dilate small arteries and reduce the production of renin, a substance known to raise blood pressure by narrowing the vessels. These are often used for patients who have had a prior heart attack. They're also often used for heart palpitations, congestive heart failure, anxiety, and glaucoma, but are generally avoided with patients who already have a slow heart rate. Common side effects include fatigue and dizziness.

4. **Calcium channel blockers**. These blockers slow down the flow of calcium into the muscle cells of the heart. This actually tones down the heart muscle contractions while also expanding the blood vessels, thereby reducing blood pressure. They can sometimes react negatively with other drugs,

however, and common side effects include fatigue, ankle swelling, and constipation.

5. **Peripherally acting drugs**. These reduce the actions of certain hormones resulting in a reduction in the speed and force of the heart's contractions. Side effects may include fatigue, dizziness, and a decrease in sexual ability. And they're sometimes avoided with elderly patients.

6. **Angiotensin II antagonists**. These medications block angiotensin II, an enzyme that raises blood pressure by promoting sodium and water retention. With a low side effect profile, they've become fairly popular and often used as an alternative to ACE inhibitors if the use of ACE inhibitors results in the development of a cough.

7. **Centrally acting alpha adrenergics**. These work on the sympathetic nervous system to reduce blood pressure, blocking the neurotransmitters that would otherwise trigger an increase in pressure. Many times these are used on an as needed basis, rather than as part of an ongoing treatment regimen. Dry mouth is a possible side effect, as is drowsiness.

BLOOD PRESSURE MEDICATIONS COME IN A VARIETY
OF BRAND NAMES. WHAT KIND OF BLOOD PRESSURE
MEDICATION IS YOURS?

FIND IT HERE:

BLOOD PRESSURE MEDICATIONS

Diuretics
Aldactazide, Aldactone, Bumex, Demadex, Diuril, Dyrenium,
Enduron, Esidrix, HydroDiuril, Hygroton, Inspra, Lasix, Lozol,
Microzide, Midamor, Mykrox, Oretic, Renese, Saluron, Thalitone,
Zaroxolyn

ACE Inhibitors
Accupril, Aceon, Altace, Capoten, Lotensin, Mavik, Monopril,
Prinivil, Uniretic, Univasc, Vasotec, Zestril

Beta blockers
Betapace, Blocadren, Bystolic, Cartrol, Coreg, Corgard, Inderal,
Inderal LA, Kerlone,Levatol, Lopressor, Normodyne, Sectral,
Tenormin, Toprol XL, Trandate, Visken, Zebeta, Ziac

Calcium channel blockers
Adalat, Adalat CC, Calan, Calan SR, Cardene SR, Cardizem CD,
Cardizem LA, Cardizem SR, Cleviprex, Covera HS, Dilacor XR,
Dynacirc CR, Isoptin, Isoptin SR, Lotrel, Norvasc, Plendil, Procardia,
Procardia XL, Sular, Tiazac, Vasocor, Verelan, Verelan PM

Peripherally acting drugs
Cardura, Dibenzyline, Minipress, Hytrin

Angiotensin II antagonists
Atacand, Avapro, Benicar, Cozaar, Diovan, Edarbi, Micardis,
Teveten

Centrally acting alpha andrenergic
Catapres, Tenex

Shyla T. High, M.D.

Medication for High Cholesterol

As we learned in Chapter Two, high cholesterol, though dangerous, can frequently be treated by lifestyle changes. Modifications to one's diet and the inclusion of exercise can dramatically reduce one's susceptibility to unsafe levels of low-density lipoprotein (LDL) cholesterol as well as triglycerides.

In many cases, however, you might need some help. And medical science has made available to us medications that are no less than life saving. Cholesterol-lowering drugs include:

1. **Statins.** Statins work in the liver to prevent the formation of cholesterol. They're effective in the lowering of LDL and triglycerides, and have even been shown to raise, modestly, the level of HDL (good cholesterol).

2. **Bile acid sequestrants**. Otherwise known as bile acid-binding drugs or simply resins, these medications go to work on the intestines, helping your body to dispose of cholesterol.

3. **Selective cholesterol absorption inhibitors**. Like bile acid sequestrants, these go to work on the intestines, too, but in a way that prevents the absorption of cholesterol.

4. **Fibric acids**. Fibric acids are typically used to reduce the level of triglycerides. They're not very effective at lowering LDL, but your doctor may recommend them once your LDL level is acceptable.

5. **Nicotinic acid**. Or simply niacin, this works in the liver (similarly to statins) but specifically to hamper the production of blood fats. Niacin can be taken as a dietary supplement.

COMMON BRAND NAMES FOR CHOLESTEROL MEDICATION
BY CATEGORY

CHOLESTEROL MEDICATIONS

Statins
Altoprev, Crestor, Lipitor, Lescol, Pravachol, Zocor

Bile acid sequestrants
Colestid, Questran, Welchol

Selective cholesterol absorption inhibitors
Zetia

Fibric acids
Lopid, Tricor

Nicotinic acid
Niacor, Niaspan

All of these have possible side effects, ranging from muscle pain to increased blood sugar levels to neurological side effects like memory loss to, in the

Shyla T. High, M.D.

case of statins specifically, potential liver damage. No matter what you're prescribed, you'll want to ask your doctor what to watch for. If you start to experience side effects, there are ways around them. Your doctor may ask you to take a break from the drug, just to confirm that what you're experiencing is, in fact, due to the medication. He or she might elect to give you a lower dose or switch to another drug. A liver enzyme test may be ordered shortly after the introduction of statins. There are supplements available that your doctor might recommend to help prevent the side effects. Don't try to address the side effects yourself. If you're feeling muscle pain, for example, don't take an over-the-counter pain reliever without first consulting your doctor.

The thing to remember is this: the potential side effects are very rarely serious and, though they may be annoying, the benefits far exceed the risk. Studies confirm that for women with cardiovascular disease, treatment of high cholesterol is effective in reducing cardiovascular events. And the data is strong that statins in particular are especially effective with secondary prevention, treating people who have already had heart attacks. Lowering your cholesterol can be life saving, and the chances of serious complications from taking cholesterol-lowering drugs are slight. In fact, when a patient voices her worries to me about the seriousness of side effects, I tell her there's more risk in the drive home from my office than in taking her cholesterol medication.

Things to Ask Your Doctor

Whether it's high blood pressure medication or cholesterol-lowering medication, your doctor will prescribe the right medication for your particular needs and circumstances. And of course that means your doctor will do a full evaluation of your health, including blood tests that will reveal potential problems (especially with your cholesterol levels). Don't be afraid to ask your doctor about the specifics of any tests he or she is doing, and to share the results with you.

In prescribing heart disease prevention medication, your doctor will take into account your overall health, your history, other conditions you may be taking medications for, and other factors that collectively will tell him or her what the best course of treatment is for you. And of course your doctor will also monitor your progress and routinely check the effectiveness of the medication(s) prescribed.

For your part, you'll want to ask your doctor exactly what you're being prescribed and why. Ask about the side effects. Make sure you know if there are other prescriptions that you're taking that ought to be avoided. Ask about over-the-counter medica-

Shyla T. High, M.D.

tions that you should avoid or if there are certain foods or beverages that you should stay away from. Make sure the prescription is okay for you if you are pregnant or nursing.

For further information about your prescribed drugs in particular, visit the FDA online. You can find a searchable, alphabetized database: www.accessdata.fda.gov/scripts/cder/drugsatfda.

Be in the Right Half

Several recent studies have found, dismayingly, that about half the people who take heart prevention medication quit taking it, typically within a year. Even among people who have had heart attacks, a full third quit taking their medication!

Reasons given are many. Cost is a factor for some. Side effects are a factor for others. Some people just don't want to take the time. One of the most common reasons is based on a dangerous misperception: the person feels fine, has no obvious symptoms of anything wrong and simply doesn't feel the need for medication. But of course this is why high blood pressure and high cholesterol are both known as *silent* killers. These insidious conditions produce very little in the way of warning signs, even as they're weakening your health and your heart. Don't wait until it's too late. According to the

American Journal of Medicine (June 27, 2012, online), 130,000 people die in the U.S. each year as a direct result of not taking their prescribed heart disease prevention medications.

Before I became a cardiologist, I was a pharmacist for years. And I know something about these medications. Trust me—if you've been prescribed heart disease prevention medication and you're not taking it, you have to start. Whatever your excuse is, find a way around it. There are a lot of things your doctor can do for you but this is one thing you can do for yourself. Along with the requisite lifestyle changes, taking your medications is *your* part of the process. You need to be an informed and active participant. No less than your life depends on it.

Pulse Points

- Whether it's for primary treatment (treatment for high risk individuals) or secondary treatment (treatment for those who have already experienced a heart event), the goal is the same: reducing your risk and lengthening your life!

- Hypertension is a silent killer that isn't under control for 70% of the adult population. But with the right medication, it's easy to manage.

- High cholesterol is another silent killer. If lifestyle changes aren't working, your doctor will prescribe the right medication for you.

- Side effects of heart disease prevention meds are minimal, low-risk, and can often be alleviated. Ask your doctor.

- Take your meds! The life you save may be your own.

Shyla T. High, M.D.

CHAPTER EIGHT

Sex, Suds, Supplements, and Stress

(The things I get asked about the most)

There are certain issues that patients ask me about regularly. They're important issues and, unfortunately, straight, simple answers aren't always available to the patient who does her own research. It seems there's an ongoing onslaught of information coming forth from the medical research community and it can be overwhelming and confusing. And the real truth is not always easily accessible. One has to deal with rumors, conflicting information, and even misleading advertising. There's a lot of noise out there and it's often difficult enough for the doctor to wade through it all, let alone the layman.

Here, however, are some straightforward answers, based on the very latest research, to four of the most pressing questions that my patients present me with.

Can I?

Of all the things I get asked about, one of the most common is sex. Namely: if I've had a heart attack, is it okay for me to resume my sex life? It's an important question. Sexual intimacy isn't something we want to have to give up. The short answer is yes, it's okay. But please ask your doctor. He or she may be concerned depending on your condition and how well you've been responding to treatment.

Generally speaking, assuming you're not experimenting by hanging off the chandeliers, sexual intercourse isn't any more physically demanding than, say, a brisk walk or routine gardening. So, if you can handle those activities without difficulty, sex should be fine, too. The fact is less than one percent of heart attacks occur during sex.

As to whether you *can* have sex—functionally, women have the advantage over men. Whereas heart disease might cause erectile dysfunction in men, no such performance dysfunction has been linked to women with heart issues.

Bottom line, get permission from your doctor and enjoy.

Should I?

It seems that if I'm not being asked about sex, I'm being asked about alcohol. There's been a lot of

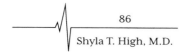

Shyla T. High, M.D.

interest in this subject ever since the discovery of the so-called French paradox. It's been noted that French people, despite having a diet relatively high in saturated fats, have a lower incidence of heart disease than Americans. The reason? Some believe it's the French people's preference for red wine. Is there something special about red wine? About alcohol in general?

Studies have found that, indeed, there may be benefits to consuming moderate amounts of alcohol. As yet, however, there's been no actual scientific link. We can't find the cause and effect, in other words. All we know is this: women who consume one or two drinks per day seem to have a reduced heart attack risk versus women who don't drink at all. But the old proverb is right on the money: in all things, moderation. More than two drinks a day and the risk increases for other problems, notably breast cancer and, naturally, diseases linked to alcohol specifically, like liver disease.

Here's your bottom line on alcohol: if you enjoy a glass of wine (or even two) a day, no problem. And a "glass", by the way, is considered to be five ounces, equivalent to a 12 ounce beer, or a 1.25 ounce (shot) of liquor. If you drink more than that, you're not doing yourself any favors and, in fact, may be doing yourself harm. If you don't drink at all, given the risk (alcohol can be addicting, after all) don't start. Have a glass of wine because you want to have a glass of wine, not because you think it might help you prevent heart disease. There are other lifestyle changes you can make for that, principally diet and exercise.

The Status on Supplements

Dietary supplements are another one of those areas that seem to produce a lot of questions. There's a lot of information out there and it's not all consistent. One problem is that medical science is still learning. One study reveals one thing, then another comes along that reveals the opposite. Here's one idea I know for sure: everything we need in order to live healthy lives can be found naturally. God gave it all to us in fruits, vegetables, and sunshine.

But just in case you feel you're not getting enough of something that you think might help you in your quest to prevent or treat heart disease, let's try to sort out the very latest information about supplements.

Calcium: Calcium supplements are often prescribed to women who have gone through menopause as a way to help keep their bones healthy. Recently, however, a controversial German study found a link associating calcium supplements with an increase in cardiovascular disease. Not calcium,

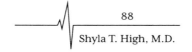

Shyla T. High, M.D.

mind you; the amount of calcium in someone's diet didn't seem to matter. The problem seemed to be the supplements. Some, however, are questioning the study, wondering whether enough other factors were taken into account. People taking calcium supplements might be in poorer health to begin with, for instance. Though the study tried to make adjustments for such factors, the study didn't pose a reason for the increase in CVD. Just like with alcohol, science has yet to find a cause-and-effect link.

Bottom line: check with your doctor. As is the case with most health issues, your *specific circumstances* may determine whether or not you should continue taking calcium supplements.

Vitamin D: I call this the sunshine vitamin. That's where you can find it naturally. The body produces most of the vitamin D a person needs as a response to sunlight. This doesn't mean you should expose yourself to harmful ultraviolet rays, of course. You can find vitamin D elsewhere, like in eggs or dairy products. For heart health, it appears to be an important vitamin. Studies show a link between low vitamin D levels and cardiovascular disease. But here's the thing: studies have also shown *no* reduction in heart disease risk by taking vitamin D supplements.

Bottom line: Don't take vitamin D supplements with any kind of expectation of decreasing your risk of cardiovascular disease.

Vitamin E: Vitamin E has attracted a lot of attention in recent years. It's a fat-soluble vitamin, meaning that it can be stored in fatty tissue. It's an antioxidant, which means that it defends cells from oxidation, a chemical process that can produce something known as "free radicals," unstable molecules in the body that seek to bond to other molecules, causing potential damage to cells or to the DNA within the cells. As far as the heart goes, it's theorized that the prevention of oxidation of LDL cholesterol might reduce plaque development. Vitamin E is also thought to reduce certain substances (prostaglandins) that cause platelet clumping, which can lead to a heart attack.

All well and good. But, as with vitamin D, all just so much theory. Studies have so far failed to show any kind of significant reduction in cardiovascular disease from the taking of vitamin E supplements. That doesn't mean that studies might not someday support doing so.

Bottom line: At this point in time, there doesn't seem to be any reason to start taking vitamin E supplements. But keep an eye on this one. There will certainly be a lot more research to come.

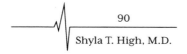

Fish Oil Supplements: Fish oil has received a lot of attention ever since it was discovered that people who regularly include oily fish in their diets (e.g., salmon, tuna, sardines), seemed to be at reduced risk for heart disease due to the presence in the fish of beneficial omega-3 fatty acids. Unfortunately, the very latest findings seem to contradict the idea that fish oil supplements make any significant difference. Although eating the fish seems to help, the supplements don't.

Bottom line: Just another example that underscores the fact that what you find in nature always seems to be better than what you find in the stores.

Miscellaneous supplements: Vitamin C, Beta-Carotene, multivitamins, and various antioxidants are other supplements that come up in discussion from time to time within the medical community, with some studies showing possible benefits but with most studies showing negligible benefits if any at all.

Bottom line: As with all supplements, if you're currently taking a supplement and it's been okayed (maybe even prescribed) by your doctor, by all means keep taking it. If you're contemplating adding a supplement for the express purpose of reducing your heart attack risk, don't bother. One important caveat: keep an eye on the latest that medical science has to offer. Research is always ongoing. A sub-caveat: don't always believe everything you read, especially if you've found it on the Internet. Research is often mischaracterized. If you have a question about the effectiveness of a supplement—or any form of treatment for that matter—check with the person who's most likely to have the very latest information: your cardiologist.

The Scoop on Stress

It might seem intuitive that stress presents a risk for heart disease. And maybe this is why I find patients often concerned about the effects of stress on their heart health. As mentioned way back in Chapter One, we have a tendency to think of the prototypical heart attack victim as being the middle-aged, stressed-out business executive. What you might find surprising, however, is that science hasn't been able to find an exact link between stress and heart disease. We don't know exactly how, in other words, stress is a factor. But enough studies have been done to assure us that it is. A recent Harvard study, in fact, found that women in highly stressful jobs are 40% more likely to develop heart disease than women in less stressful occupations.[3]

---

[3] http://www.health.harvard.edu/press_releases/research-uncovers-strong-link-between-work-related-stress-and-heart-problems

Shyla T. High, M.D.

There's no reason to wait for science to discover the precise link on this one. It might be that stress hormones, speeding up the blood rate and constricting blood vessels, may do long-term damage to the cardiovascular system. It might also be that stressed individuals might be more apt to lead unhealthy lives, exercising little and eating poorly. But whatever the link, it's there and it cannot be ignored.

If you often feel that you're living a pressure-packed life, consider making the time (you can find it) to do things to help mitigate your stress. Exercise reduces anxiety. Meditation and other relaxation techniques can also help bring about some healthy peace of mind. Seek some kind of outlet. Find some quiet time away from the cares of the world. Taking care of your mental health turns out to be significantly important for your physical well-being, too.

Pulse Points

🔹 Sex after a heart attack is normally okay. But check with your doctor just to make certain it's okay for you in particular.

🔹 One or two servings of alcohol a day is acceptable. But no more. And if you don't drink at all, there's no need to start.

- There's little reason to begin taking supplements for the purpose of treating your heart disease. If you insist, however, at least get your doctor's opinion.

- Stress can be a killer. If you find yourself feeling under pressure a lot of the time, start looking for ways to relax.

CHAPTER NINE

Other Heart Conditions

A Working Machine

Rightfully so, coronary artery disease and atherosclerosis get most of the headlines, most of everybody's attention. Heart failure is a scary thing. But there are other heart conditions, too—other things that can go wrong with the heart, some serious, some not so serious.

The heart, after all, is a working machine and machines sometimes develop problems. There are several parts of the heart machine that have to operate together and function properly at all times. It might seem complex, but it's really pretty simple. There's a plumbing system (arteries) and a pump (ventricles) and an electrical system and four valves and a lining. And when they all work together, it's a beautiful thing. When they don't, we need to figure out what's wrong. We need to figure out what part of the machine isn't doing its job.

We've learned about the big issues; now let's take a look at some of the smaller ones.

Your Murmuring Heart

A heart murmur is just what you might think—a sound the heart makes. Typically, the sound represents the blood flowing through the heart in a turbulent, uneven way. You won't be able to hear it yourself; murmurs are most commonly detected by a physician's stethoscope during a physical examination.

A heart murmur can be caused by a number of factors including abnormalities of the valves (more on this in a bit), the presence of a small hole in the wall between the heart's chambers, and congenital defects (from birth, which often self-correct). Most murmurs are completely benign but your doctor may want to investigate further. He or she might order an echocardiogram (the test we discussed in Chapter Four that is essentially a sonogram of the heart), providing the doctor with a picture from which he or she can ascertain the root cause of the murmur.

Treatment will depend on what the doctor finds. Serious cases of structural damage might progress until they ultimately require surgery to repair or replace a valve. Sometimes a murmur might be caused by an infection which will require antibiotics. Many times a murmur might just be a harmless, life-long condition requiring nothing more than occasional monitoring.

Valvular Disorders

Your heart has four valves that open to allow blood to flow through the chambers and shut to keep it from flowing backwards. When they work the way they're supposed to, assuming everything else is functioning properly, the blood moves smoothly and unidirectionally. But sometimes a valve may not close properly, or maybe not open fully. This can prevent the proper flow of blood and/or lead to backflow.

Symptoms can include palpitations, dizziness, and shortness of breath. Or you might experience vague symptoms such as generalized weakness or chest discomfort. Your doctor may hear a murmur, as discussed above, and order an echocardiogram

Valve problems are remarkably common. Like murmurs, some of them are congenital in nature. Others—degenerative valve disorders—appear with age. Some require nothing but occasional moni-toring, others require treatment. Your doctor will make the determination.

Medications for ongoing valve disorders can help to some degree, at least with the symptoms, but more serious cases might require corrective surgery.

Electrical Abnormalities

We talked a little about heart palpitations in Chapter Five and how they can sometimes provide a sense of chest pressure or discomfort, leading to the idea that you're having a heart attack. But even without the pressure and discomfort, even with just an extra beat or a fluttering rhythm, I have found that heart palpitations can be scary for many people. It's understandable; it's disconcerting to think that something is interfering with the regular beating of your heart.

And yet, heart palpitations are almost always harmless. Most of the time the problem is specific to the electrical system and not reflective of other issues, such as serious blockage.

We can think of electrical abnormalities as being in one of two major categories, both falling under the general term arrhythmia. The first is experienced as extra beats, originating in either the top chamber (left or right atrium), called premature atrial contractions (PACs), or in the lower chamber (left

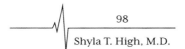

or right ventricle), called premature ventricle contractions (PVCs). These are often described by patients as "thumps" or "flip-flop" sensations. Often, rather than feeling the extra beat, a patient might feels as though a beat has been skipped. This kind of arrhythmia may be caused by such things as nicotine, caffeine, stress, or intense physical exertion. Sometimes the cause might be hormonal changes due to pregnancy or menopause (and sometimes menstruation.) Irritating, though benign, symptoms of this kind of heart palpitation can often be alleviated with medication. But sometimes the side effects of the medication can be worse than the palpitations. In most cases, it's better to identify the source and work on that end of the problem. In other words, reduce the nicotine or caffeine or stress or physical exertion. Frequently, absent no treatment at all, the condition will go away with the passage of time.

The second category of heart palpitations is experienced as more of a flutter or racing heart. This is usually a fast rhythm that originates from the top chamber of the heart, most commonly atrial fibrillation or atrial flutter. Or, sometimes, from just above the ventricles, called supraventricular tachycardia. As with extra heart beats, a fast rhythm is frequently benign. Atrial fibrillation specifically can sometimes be a cause of concern, however. If blood isn't being pumped out of the atria completely, it's possible it might collect, coagulate, and present the danger of a stroke. This is a case where medication may be necessary, not just to alleviate some uncomfortable symptoms, but to reduce the risk of something worse.

To determine the proper course of action for your atrial fibrillation, your doctor will most likely use a predictive tool knows as the CHADS score. He or she will consider whether you have **C**ongestive **h**eart failure, **H**ypertension, your **A**ge, if you have **D**iabetes, and if you've had a prior **S**troke. The scoring works like this:

Congestive Heart Disease.................. 1 point

Hypertension...................................... 1 point

Age (Over 75)..................................... 1 point

Diabetes.. 1 point

Prior Stroke.. 2 points

Added together, the doctor makes his or her recommendation. A score of zero typically requires no treatment for atrial fibrillation, or perhaps maybe an aspirin taken daily. A score of 1 might require an aspirin a day or a stronger blood thinner. A score of 2 or above, signifying moderate to high risk, definitely means the prescribing of a blood-thinning agent.

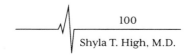

Shyla T. High, M.D.

Congestive Heart Failure

We talked about congestive heart failure above as a factor helping to determine a doctor's course of action with atrial fibrillation. In fact, we've mentioned congestive heart failure a few times in this book, and it's a term that you often hear within discussions about the heart. But what, exactly, is it?

In the simplest terms, congestive heart failure describes a condition wherein the heart simply isn't functioning adequately to do its job pumping the blood. The cause can be a myriad of things. Congestive heart failure is an umbrella term, in other words. People are said to die of congestive heart failure, and while that's technically true, it's really the end result of other, underlying causes.

If you've been diagnosed with congestive heart failure, your doctor is going to determine the underlying cause. It can be from elevated blood pressure, coronary artery disease (with its own set of causes), valve disorders, infections, or other conditions. Once the cause is identified, then the appropriate treatment can begin. Individuals with congestive heart failure, properly treated, can often lead normal, active, productive lives.

One treatment option, especially appropriate for a heart that has become weakened to the point of potentially life-threatening rhythm abnormality, is the insertion of an implantable cardioverter-defibrillator (ICD). An ICD is a small, thin, battery-powered device that is permanently implanted underneath the skin just outside the ribcage. Its purpose is to detect dangerous rhythm abnormalities, at which point it will deliver a small jolt of electricity, thus getting the heart back to normal rhythm. The ICD is an amazing and effective piece of modern technology.

Pericarditis

Like palpitations, and as we touched on in Chapter Five, pericarditis can mimic heart attack pain. But it's a problem not with the electrical system or the plumbing system, but with the lining of the heart—the pericardium. It's an inflammation, caused by a viral or bacterial infection. It may be the result of the flu or even a bad cold. Frequently you might never even learn what the original cause was.

You'll feel pericarditis as chest pain when you take a deep breath, or maybe move your upper body in a certain way. Anti-inflammatory medications are typically sufficient for treatment and some cases go away on their own.

Pulse Points

- Cardiovascular disease isn't the only thing that can go wrong with the heart. As with any machine, a part here or there can create problems—some more serious than others.

- Heart murmurs are typically benign, but your doctor will investigate to make sure.

- Valve disorders can create problems with the flow of blood through the heart. Degenerative ones can be serious and need to be treated not unlike coronary artery disease.

- Heart palpitations resulting from electrical problems are very rarely serious, but if your atrial fibrillation presents a risk due to other conditions, your doctor will want to prescribe treatment.

- Congestive heart failure is more or less a symptom of a serious underlying cause that requires serious treatment.

- Pericarditis is an inflammation of the lining of the heart and easily treatable with antibiotics.

CHAPTER TEN

Leftovers

By now, you should have a pretty good handle
on heart health—heart attack risk, heart attack
symptoms, heart attack prevention, other heart
conditions, testing and diagnostic procedures, treatments, meds, supplements, what you can do, what
you can't do, etc. And maybe all your questions have
been answered.

But the heart (the human body for that matter)
is a rather involved piece of machinery. It seems
we're learning more and more about it every day.
And what we know is so plentiful, it doesn't necessarily fit neatly into categories that can be sectioned
off into formal chapters. Some of it spills over. It's a
smorgasbord of information. You try to take it all
in, but inevitably there's a plate or two of leftovers.
Herewith, then, some additional things for you to
chew on, important things that I didn't want to leave
out.

105

Aspirin

There always seems to be a lot of discussion about aspirin where the heart is concerned. It's a blood thinning agent, of course, and can be a key for the treatment of heart disease. But not always. The question is, is it right for you? The short answer? Ask your doctor.

A more comprehensive answer involves these very latest guidelines from the U.S. Preventive Services Task Force (USPSTF): Given the risk of gastrointestinal hemorrhage (aspirin has been known to cause stomach bleeding), the daily use of aspirin is recommended if 1) you're between the ages of 55 and 79, and 2) the benefit of aspirin in reducing your risk of stroke (from such underlying causes as CVD, hypertension, diabetes, smoking, and atrial fibrillation) outweighs the risk. Under 55? Over 80? In both cases, the USPSTF recommends *against* aspirin. So, if you're somewhere between 55 and 79, and you have a condition or conditions that may put you at risk for stroke, consider the daily use of aspirin. (Check with your doctor first, of course). Otherwise, maybe keep it handy for the occasional headache.

Shyla T. High, M.D.

Coffee

Coffee is a subject that has been mired in conflicting information over the years. Is it good for the heart? Is it bad? Is it neutral? One of the problems medical researchers have with something as complex as the human being (and this hold true for any serious medical research), is that there are often too many other variables to take into account; too many to allow for.

For example, the very latest research on coffee, a study of close to 200,000 women between the ages of 50 and 71 over the course of 13 years[4] initially revealed a correlation between coffee and risk of death. But then the researchers noticed that many of the people in the study smoked, as well as drank coffee. In fact, those who drank coffee were more likely to smoke than those who didn't drink coffee. When the researchers adjusted their findings to take into account the risk from smoking, the risk from coffee was actually shown to be of an *inverse* relationship. Coffee drinkers were less likely to die of heart disease, respiratory disease, and stroke, compared with non coffee drinkers. And that seemed to hold true for up to six cups of coffee per day!

So that's the very latest on coffee. But here's

---

[4] "Association of Coffee Drinking with Total and Cause-Specific Mortality", Freedman, Park, et al, New England Journal of Medicine, May 17, 2012.

another problem medical researchers often face. Doing a study on a group of people (even a large group of people) doesn't tell the researchers *why* a given finding is true. We don't know why drinking coffee seems to lower the risk of heart disease, for example. We're not sure of the connection.

And so, as with alcohol, if you're not drinking coffee, I don't think there's really a reason, heart-health-wise, to start. But if you're drinking coffee, I see no reason to stop.

Hormones and Heart Health

Exogenous hormones—hormones introduced (usually orally) as either contraceptives or for hormone-replacement therapy—seem to present some potential problems. But just how big is that potential? As with anything related to the human body, introducing something extra can have unintended consequences. Everything is interrelated. Supplemental hormones like estrogen have been shown to raise the risk of blood clots, leading to stroke. The data on heart disease is less clear, but there does seem to be a connection between oral contraceptives and high cholesterol and hypertension. But this connection is not a strong one. And much weaker than it was in the early days of contraception. The pill is simply safer now.

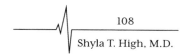

Shyla T. High, M.D.

With all that said, the risk seems to be higher (unsurprisingly) for women who smoke or have other risk factors, like pre-existing hypertension or obesity or diabetes, etc. So, if you don't smoke and you're healthy with no other risk factors, exogenous hormones are probably just fine for you. As always, check with your doctor first.

Depression

Have you experienced a heart attack? We doctors have a way of focusing almost entirely on physical health when it comes to secondary prevention—treating someone who's had a heart attack to make sure she doesn't have another one. Too often, we ignore the individual's mental health. But depression is a real problem for heart patients, with up to a third experiencing some form of it. Certainly it's understandable; someone who's had a heart attack has been forced to come face to face with her very mortality.

Studies show that people who suffer from depression after a cardiac event are more likely to have another cardiac event. (Which, of course, is even *more* depressing.) We're not really sure of the reason. Depression, in and of itself, may not be the real culprit. The higher risk of a second heart attack might be because depressed people have a greater tendency to do unhealthy things. They may smoke more or eat more fattening foods or exercise less (or not at all).

Are you depressed? Symptoms can include losing interest in activities you used to enjoy, frequent crying for no specific reason, feelings of sluggishness, not sleeping well or getting too much sleep, negative thoughts, even thoughts of suicide. If any of this sounds familiar, you need to bring it to your doctor's attention. There's no reason to suffer with depression. Take care of yourself—emotionally as well as physically. Lots of people have heart attacks and live full, happy, long lives. You can, too.

Happy People, Happy Hearts

Speaking of mental health, whether you've experienced a heart attack or not, what you probably already know intuitively is, indeed, true: people who are generally happier about life seem to have a lower risk of heart disease. Stressed people, on the other hand, are much more at risk. You already know from Chapter Eight that, according to a recent study, women in highly stressful jobs are 40% more likely to develop heart disease than women in less stressful occupations. But in another recent study[5], researchers found that people who work 11 or more

---

[5] "Using Additional Information on Working Hours to Predict Coronary Heart Disease - A Cohort Study", Kivimäki, Mika, et al, *Annals of Internal Medicine* April 4, 2011 vol. 154 no. 7 457-463

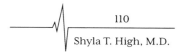

hours a day have an astounding 67% greater chance of developing heart disease than their less workaholic counterparts. Extra hours frequently mean more stress, less exercise, and poorer eating habits. And more than one study has revealed that people who generally regard themselves as optimists—glass half-full people as opposed to glass half-empty people—have a reduced risk of dying from heart disease as well as a host of other diseases. The lesson seems clear: smile more, worry less, and live longer.

And while you're looking for ways to stay happy, here's a simple thing you can do that might make you smile even as it directly helps your heart: pump up the jams. It's been shown that listening to music increases blood flow and relaxes the cardiovascular system. Find yourself thirty uninterrupted minutes a day to listen to the music of your choice.

Pay Attention

A final word of advice. You've taken a big step towards a healthy heart just by reading this book. And if you follow the guidelines and suggestions herein, you're going to minimize your risk of cardiovascular disease and/or a second heart attack. But it doesn't end here. Keep learning and keep yourself informed. I have found in my practice that the more educated a patient is about her health, the healthier she is. That's no coincidence.

So pay attention to the information that's out there. It's not always easy. The Internet is a virtual fire hose of it, and you don't always know what to believe and what not to believe. There are some trusted sources, however. The American Heart Association is one (www.heart.org). Your own doctor is another. It's his or her job to keep up with the latest developments and to make sure you're getting the testing and treatment you need.

By keeping yourself informed, you'll be taking a monumental step towards good heart health. Remember this from Chapter One: 75% of heart disease is preventable! In a world where it seems as though circumstances are often beyond our control, heart health doesn't have to be one of those things. It really is up to *you*.

So stay alert and pay attention. And may you live a long, happy, heart-healthy life!

Shyla T. High, M.D.

Pulse Points

- As a potential avenue for heart disease treatment, aspirin may be considered if you're between the ages of 55 and 79 and you're at heart disease risk.

- Are you a coffee drinker? There's no reason to stop. Enjoy.

- Your birth control pills are most likely fine so long as you're not in a high risk group for cardiovascular disease.

- Depression after a heart attack is common. But it can also present a serious obstacle to becoming well. If you're depressed, talk to your doctor.

- Don't worry, be happy, and live longer.

- Keep informed. We're learning new things all the time!

APPENDIX I

BMI Chart

	Normal						Overweight					Obese									Extreme Obesity															
	19	20	21	22	23	24	25	26	27	28	29	30	31	32	33	34	35	36	37	38	39	40	41	42	43	44	45	46	47	48	49	50	51	52	53	54
Height (inches)	Body Weight (pounds)																																			
	91	96	100	105	110	115	119	124	129	134	138	143	148	153	158	162	167	172	177	181	186	191	196	201	205	210	215	220	224	229	234	239	244	248	253	258
	94	99	104	109	114	119	124	128	133	138	143	148	153	158	163	168	173	178	183	188	193	198	203	208	212	217	222	227	232	237	242	247	252	257	262	267
	97	102	107	112	118	123	128	133	138	143	148	153	158	163	168	174	179	184	189	194	199	204	209	215	220	225	230	235	240	245	250	255	261	266	271	276
	100	106	111	116	122	127	132	137	143	148	153	158	164	169	174	180	185	190	195	201	206	211	217	222	227	232	238	243	248	254	259	264	269	275	280	285
	104	109	115	120	126	131	136	142	147	153	158	164	169	175	180	186	191	196	202	207	213	218	224	229	235	240	246	251	256	262	267	273	278	284	289	295
	107	113	118	124	130	135	141	146	152	158	163	169	175	180	186	191	197	203	208	214	220	225	231	237	242	248	254	259	265	270	278	282	287	293	299	304
	110	116	122	128	134	140	145	151	157	163	169	174	180	186	192	197	204	209	215	221	227	232	238	244	250	256	262	267	273	279	285	291	296	302	308	314
	114	120	126	132	138	144	150	156	162	168	174	180	186	192	198	204	210	216	222	228	234	240	246	252	258	264	270	276	282	288	294	300	306	312	318	324
	118	124	130	136	142	148	155	161	167	173	179	186	192	198	204	210	216	223	229	235	241	247	253	260	266	272	278	284	291	297	303	309	315	322	328	334
	121	127	134	140	146	153	159	166	172	178	185	191	198	204	211	217	223	230	236	242	249	255	261	268	274	280	287	293	299	306	312	319	325	331	338	344
	125	131	138	144	151	158	164	171	177	184	190	197	203	210	216	223	230	236	243	249	256	262	269	276	282	289	295	302	308	315	322	328	335	341	348	354
	128	135	142	149	155	162	169	176	182	189	196	203	209	216	223	230	236	243	250	257	263	270	277	284	291	297	304	311	318	324	331	338	345	351	358	365
	132	139	146	153	160	167	174	181	188	195	202	209	216	222	229	236	243	250	257	264	271	278	285	292	299	306	313	320	327	334	341	348	355	362	369	376
	136	143	150	157	165	172	179	186	193	200	208	215	222	229	236	243	250	257	265	272	279	286	293	301	308	315	322	329	338	343	351	358	365	372	379	386
	140	147	154	162	169	177	184	191	199	206	213	221	228	235	242	250	258	265	272	279	287	294	302	309	316	324	331	338	346	353	361	368	375	383	390	397
	144	151	159	166	174	182	189	197	204	212	219	227	235	242	250	257	265	272	280	288	295	302	310	318	325	333	340	348	355	363	371	378	386	393	401	408
	148	155	163	171	179	186	194	202	210	218	225	233	241	249	256	264	272	280	287	295	303	311	319	326	334	342	350	358	365	373	381	389	396	404	412	420
	152	160	168	176	184	192	200	208	216	224	232	240	248	256	264	272	279	287	295	303	311	319	327	335	343	351	359	367	375	383	391	399	407	415	423	431
	156	164	172	180	189	197	205	213	221	230	238	246	254	263	271	279	287	295	304	312	320	328	336	344	353	361	369	377	385	394	402	410	418	426	435	443

Why Most Women Die

Shyla T. High, M.D.

A

abnormal rhythm, 59, 98–100
ACE inhibitors, 73–74, 76
acid reflux, 53–54
activity, 17–19, 34
acute coronary syndrome (ACS), 62
African-American women, 2
alcohol consumption, 86–88
allergies, 60
ambulance transport, 59–60
angina pectoris, 12–13, 38–39, 62
angiogram, 62–64
angiography, 45
angioplasty, 61, 64–66
angiotensin converting enzymes (ACE) inhibitors, 73–74, 76
angiotensin II antagonists, 75–76
antioxidants, 90
anxiety, 55–56, 92–93, 110–111
aortic dissection, 49–50
arrhythmia, 59, 98–100
arterial blockage, 12–13, 38, 39, 64–67
aspirin, 60, 100, 106
atherosclerosis, 11
atherosclerotic vascular disease, 11
atrial fibrillation, 99–100
awareness, 8–10

B

bacterial infections, 51
balloon angioplasty, 61, 64–66
beta blockers, 74, 76
bile acid sequestrants, 77–78
blocked arteries, 12–13, 38, 39, 64–67

blood clots, 13, 54–55, 60, 61, 65, 108
blood pressure, high, 16, 17, 19–22, 50, 72–76, 81–82
Bloom, David, 55
body mass index (BMI), 18, 115
breathing cessation, 60–61
bypass surgery, 66–68

C

calcium channel blockers, 74–76
calcium score, 45
calcium supplements, 88–89
cardiac catheterization, 62–64
cardiac enzyme tests, 61
cardio CT scan, 45
cardiopulmonary resuscitation (CPR), 60–61
cardiovascular disease (CVD). *See* heart disease
centrally acting alpha adrenergics, 75–76
CHADS score, 100
chemically replicated stress test, 43
chest pain
   angina, 12–13, 38–39, 62
   cardiac, 49–52
   causes and symptoms, 37–38
   non-cardiac, 52–56
   treatment of, 56
cholesterol, 16, 17, 22–24, 77–80, 81
clogged vessels, 12–13, 38, 39, 64–67
clot busting medications, 61–62
clots, 13, 54–55, 60, 61, 65, 108
coffee consumption, 107–108

117

collapsed lungs, 54
computerized tomographic (CT) scan, 45
congestive heart failure, 2, 101–102
coronary artery spasms, 51–52
costochondritis, 52–53
CPR (cardiopulmonary resuscitation), 60–61
CT angiography (CTA test), 45
CVD (cardiovascular disease). *See* heart disease

D

deep vein thrombosis (DVT), 55
depression, 109–110
diabetes, 24–25
diastolic pressure, 20
diet, 19, 30–33
dietary supplements, 88–92
disconnect among women, 1–3
diuretics, 73, 76
DVT (deep vein thrombosis), 55

E

eating healthy, 19, 30–33
echocardiogram, 43
electrical abnormalities, 59, 98–100
electrocardiogram (EKG), 40–42
emergency action plan, 59–61
enzymes, 61
estrogen, 14, 108–109
exercise, 17–19, 34
exercise stress test, 39–40
exogenous hormones, 108–109

F

family history of heart disease, 14

fast heart rhythm, 99–100
fibric acids, 78
fish oil supplements, 90
free radicals, 90

G

gall bladder problems, 53–54
gastroesophageal reflux disease (GERD), 53–54
gender-based differences, 1–9, 68–69

H

HDL (high-density lipoproteins), 22–23
healthy living choices, 19, 29–36
heart attacks. *See also* heart disease
    action plan, 59–61
    defined, 13, 37
    diagnostic assessments, 61–63
    emergency room procedures, 61
    gender differences in diagnosing, 3–6, 68–69
    medications, 60, 61, 100, 106
    preventing, 69, 71–72
    sexual intimacy and, 86
    symptoms, 3–5, 13, 37–39
    treatments, 61, 64–69
heart disease. *See also* heart attacks
    defined, 11
    dietary supplements and, 88–92
    gender differences in diagnosis and treatment of, 1–9, 68–69
    happiness and, 110–111
    hormones and, 108–109
    medications for. *See* medications
    non-modifiable risk factors, 13–14

Shyla T. High, M.D.

preventing. *See*
preventing heart disease
race-based diagnostic
differences, 2, 68–69
reducing risk, 29–36
risk factors. *See* risk
factors for heart disease
screening tests, 44–46
symptom assessment
tests, 39–44
symptoms, 2–3
heart failure, 2, 101–102
heart murmurs, 96–97
heart palpitations, 52, 59, 98–100
heartbeats, irregular, 59, 98–100
heartburn, 53–54
high blood pressure, 16, 17, 19–22, 50, 72–76, 81–82
high cholesterol levels, 16, 17, 22–24, 81
high-density lipoproteins (HDL), 22–23
Hispanic-American women, 2
hormones, 52, 99
hypertension, 16, 17, 19–22, 50, 81–82

I

implantable cardioverter-defibrillator (ICD), 101–102
inactivity, 17–19
indigestion, 38
infections, 51
informed, staying, 111–112
irregular heartbeats, 59, 98–100

J

jaw pain, 39

L

LDL (low-density lipoproteins), 22, 23
lifestyle choices, 29–36

M

medications
aspirin, 60, 100, 106
blood pressure lowering, 21–22, 72–76
cholesterol lowering, 77–80
keeping a list of, 60
platelet formation reducing, 65
platelet formation reduction, 60
questioning your doctor about, 80–81
side effects, 73–75, 78–80, 106
taking as prescribed, 81–82
thrombolytics, 61–62
metabolic syndrome, 25–26
Mexican-American women, 2
M.I. (myocardial infarction). *See* heart attacks
modifiable risk factors, 15–26, 29–35
mortality rates, 1
murmurs, heart, 96–97
musculoskeletal causes of chest pain, 52–53
music, 111
myocardial infarction (M.I.). *See* heart attacks

N

nausea, 13
neck pain, 39
negative stress test result, 40
new onset angina, 62
niacin, 78
nicotinic acid, 78
non-modifiable risk factors, 14
nuclear stress test, 42–43
nutrition, 19, 30–33. *See also* dietary supplements

O

obesity, 17–19, 30–34
optimism, 111
oral contraceptives, 108–109

P

PACs (premature atrial
   contractions), 98–99
palpitations, 52, 59, 98–100
pancreatitis, 53–54
panic disorders, 55–56
pericarditis, 51, 102
peripherally acting drugs,
   75–76
physical activity, 17–19, 34
plaque buildup, 11–12, 44–46
platelets, 60
Plavix, 65
pleurisy, 51, 54
positive stress test result, 40
post-menopausal women,
   40–42
pre-hypertension, 20
premature atrial contrac-
   tions (PACs), 98–99
premature ventricle contractions (PVCs), 98–99
pressure in chest. See chest
   pain
preventing heart disease. See
   also risk factors for heart
   disease
   awareness and, 9–10
   exercise, 17–19, 34
   healthy eating, 19, 30–33.
      See also dietary supple-
      ments
   lifestyle choices, 29–36
   medications for. See
      medications
primary prevention, 71
procedures for treating heart
   attacks, 61–67
prototypical heart attack
   victim, 2
psychological causes of chest
   pain, 55–56

pulmonary embolisms, 54–
   55
PVCs (premature ventricle
   contractions), 98–99

R

race-based differences, 2,
   68–69
radiating pain in upper
   body, 39
respiratory causes of chest
   pain, 54–55
resuscitation, 60–61
rhythm abnormality, 59, 98–
   100
risk factors for heart disease.
   See also preventing heart
   disease
   alcohol consumption, 86–
      88
   coffee consumption, 107–
      108
   depression, 109–110
   diabetes, 24–25
   gender-based differences,
      1–9
   high blood pressure, 16, 17,
      19–22, 50, 81–82
   high cholesterol, 16, 17, 22–
      24, 81
   intertwined risk factors,
      25–26
   modifiable, 15–26, 29–35
   non-modifiable, 14
   obesity, 17–19, 30–34
   physical inactivity, 17–19
   race-based differences, 2
   reducing risk, 29–36
   silent killers, 20–21, 22, 81–
      82
   smoking, 7, 15–17, 30
   stress, 55–56, 92–93, 110–111
Ritter, John, 50

S

screening tests, 44–46
secondary prevention, 71

selective cholesterol absorption inhibitors, 77–78
silent killers, 20–21, 22, 81–82
smoking, 7, 15–17, 30
sonogram, 43
spasms, coronary artery, 51–52
stable angina, 38
statins, 77–79
stents, 64–66
stopped heart, 60–61
stress, 55–56, 92–93, 110–111
stress tests, 39–44, 62
strokes, 11, 19, 99–100, 106, 108–109
supplemental hormones, 108–109
supraventricular tachycardia, 99–100
sweating, 13, 38–39
symptom assessment tests, 37–44
systolic pressure, 20

T

tear in aorta wall lining, 49–50
tests
    cardiac enzyme, 61
    chemically replicated stress test, 43
    cholesterol level, 23–24
    CT angiography (CTA test), 45
    exercise stress test, 39–40
    nuclear stress test, 42–43
    screening tests, 44–46
    stress tests, 39–44, 62
    symptom assessment tests, 39–44
thrombolytics, 61–62
tightness in chest. See chest pain
triglycerides, 23, 24

U

ulcers, 53–54
unstable angina, 38–39, 62

V

valvular disorders, 97–98
vascular disease, 11
viral infections, 51
vitamin D, 89–90
vitamin E, 90

W

water pills, 73, 76
weight distribution, 18. See also obesity

Why Most Women Die

CPSIA information can be obtained at www.ICGtesting.com
Printed in the USA
BVOW011838110213

312966BV00001B/15/P